Prognosis in Musculoskeletal Injury

A handbook for doctors and lawyers

Eurig Jeffreys, FRCS(Ed.), FRCS(Eng.)
Consultant Orthopaedic Surgeon, The Robert Jones and Agnes Hunt Orthopaedic Hospital, Oswestry, and The Wrexham Maelor Hospital

BUTTERWORTH
HEINEMANN

Butterworth–Heinemann Ltd
Halley Court, Jordan Hill, Oxford OX2 8EJ

PART OF REED INTERNATIONAL P.L.C.

OXFORD LONDON GUILDFORD BOSTON MUNICH NEWDELHI SINGAPORE SYDNEY TOKYO TORONTO WELLINGTON

First published 1991

British Library Cataloguing in Publication Data

Jeffreys, Eurig
Prognosis in musculoskeletal injury.
1. Man. Musculoskeletal system. Injuries
I. Title
617.47044

ISBN 0-7506-1246-0

Library of Congress Cataloging-in-Publication Data applied for

Composition by Genesis Typesetting, Laser Quay, Rochester, Kent
Printed and bound in Great Britain by Courier International Ltd, Tiptree, Essex

Preface

The idea for this book emerged from a conversation with my colleagues when we agreed there was a need for an easily accessible reference source for prognosis following injury. Prognosis must be inexact, of necessity, because it applies to the individual the results of the many. All that a surgeon can do is to apply the principle of the balance of probabilities as demonstrated in the available literature and his own experience.

I have reviewed the relevant literature, summarized the results and presented them in tabular form. I have tried to avoid being anecdotal and to suppress any personal opinions except where they are based on published evidence. I have not dealt with head injuries, injury to the spinal cord or injury to the skin as I do not believe an orthopaedic surgeon is competent to pronounce on those subjects.

I hope the book will be useful to orthopaedic surgeons, consultants in accident medicine, doctors sitting on appeal tribunals, and to lawyers involved with personal injury litigation.

T.E.J.
Wrexham
Oswestry 1990

Acknowledgements

It gives me pleasure to acknowledge the advice and encouragement of Dr Geoffrey Smaldon, Managing Editor of Butterworth–Heinemann. It is with gratitude and affection that I record my debt to Christine Watkins, my loyal amanuensis for so many years.

Contents

Introduction

Prognosis is the forecast of the probable course of a case of disease or injury, or it is the art of making such a forecast (*Shorter Oxford English Dictionary,* 1977). These definitions emphasize three particular aspects of prognosis. It is an art, or skill, not a science. It concerns probabilities, not certainties, and it refers to the individual not the general. It follows that any attempt to reduce it to certainty by referring to proportions in series of patients will fail. Fortunately, although individuals differ in their response to insult, their ailments follow recognized patterns and it is possible to form general predictions of the natural history of disorders. Each clinician draws on his own knowledge of past cases, and modifies or confirms that knowledge by the prospective observation of each new case. Some conditions are too uncommon for one clinician to draw on personal knowledge for guidance, and he then has to rely on the published experience of others. Some clinicians, by virtue of declaring or demonstrating a special interest, accumulate a greater personal experience of a condition or group of conditions, and their knowledge of the natural history of that condition then becomes authoritative. Future historians, noting the general introduction of audit into our hospitals, will mourn the lost opportunities of the first forty years of the National Health Service, when data could have been accumulated to provide definite answers concerning the outcome of treatment.

An alternative definition of prognosis, then, could be the application of the knowledge of the natural history of a disorder in a group of people to the forecast of the behaviour of that disorder in a given individual. To a very great degree, that knowledge is available from epidemiological studies and from prospective and retrospective reports of individual conditions. However, the individual will always react in an individual way; one man's deformity is not necessarily another man's disability.

The first essential in any prognosis is accurate diagnosis, and the orthopaedic surgeon owes much in this respect to modern methods of imaging.

The second is to recognize the existence of any factors relating to that diagnosis which modify the behaviour of the lesion in question. In injury, such factors may be: the nature of the injury itself; whether it was produced by severe or moderate violence; whether the injured tissue was normal or abnormal at the time; the patient's age, diathesis, sex and occupation.

The third is to understand the effects, if any, of treatment on natural history. Treatment is a complication of natural history, which may have benign or malign effect. It has less influence on natural history than doctors like to think. In few disorders can prognosis be reversed. (I dressed him, God cured him – Ambroise Paré.)

The fourth is to consider what effect the prophesied end result will have on the patient's life. Terms to describe the residual effects of that end result are used loosely and often interchangeably. In this book the following terms will be used to describe an end result which has left the patient less perfect than before the injury occurred. They are drawn from the *WHO Classification of Disability* (1980). An *impairment* is any loss of abnormality of psychological, physiological or anatomical structure or function. A *disability* is any restriction, or lack of ability, to perform an activity in the manner of, or within the range considered normal for, a human being. A *handicap* is a disadvantage for a given individual, resulting from an impairment or disability, that limits or prevents the fulfillment of a role, depending on age, sex, social and cultural factors, for that individual.

The terms have been slightly modified in this book. Impairment has been subdivided into *structural impairment* and *subjective impairment*. Structural defects in themselves may not be a cause of symptoms. Symptoms may exist without any detectable structural fault. Both forms of impairment may singly or together contribute to a disability. They differ in that one is measurable, the other not.

Disability and handicap are relative terms, peculiar to a given individual or to a given occupation. Assessment of residual disability must also be relative, and can only be expressed in relative terms. It is for the courts, not doctors, to translate those relative terms into precise financial compensation.

Variations in the natural history of a disorder may arise from the development of complications. These may be foreseen and recognized as inevitable consequences of the injury. Their incidence will be modified by the presence of known variations in individual make up, or by the presence of anatomical peculiarities of the injured part (such as the entry of a nutrient artery). The commonest cause of any complication is treatment, in as much as treatment tries to modify natural history.

It is therefore unlikely that any prognosis will be completely accurate in any individual, even although all injured tissue must obey the laws of chemistry and physics.

The sources of impairment, disability or handicap will vary. They will include:

1. *Pain* which is not a structural impairment but can cause disability or handicap.
2. *Loss of part,* such as in amputation which is always an impairment and a disability but not necessarily a handicap.
3. *Discrepancy in limb length,* which is always an impairment, but not necessarily a disability or a handicap.
4. *Deformity,* which is an impairment but may not cause disability or handicap.
5. *Swelling* which is an impairment but not necessarily a source of disability or handicap.
6. *Restricted movement* which is an impairment, causes disability but may not constitute a handicap.

Any residuum which falls short of normality is an impairment. Impairment may have been present before the injury, such as an osteoarthrotic joint which is injured. Whether impairment inflicts disability or imposes a handicap on a given individual is variable. An impairment may result in handicap for certain activities but not for others, for work but not for leisure, or, of increasing importance in Western society, for leisure but not for work.

In the management of the injured patient a knowledge of natural history affects decisions of treatment. The surgeon's aim is to obtain as near perfect an anatomical and functional result as is consistent with the injury. Knowledge of the possible end result and its effect on the patient's life will temper decisions of interference. That is the function and importance of prognosis to the surgeon.

The lawyer has different expectations. He expects precise definitions and forecasts so that he can assess the end result in financial terms. The surgeon may be able to forecast an impairment precisely, but he will not be able to define any resulting disability or handicap as precisely as his lawyer would wish. The lawyer should understand this, and usually does. The surgeon's prognosis will be reinforced in authority if he can refer to published work, ideally his own. Lawyers recognize and respect precedent.

Even so, it must be recognized by doctor, lawyer and patient that a prognosis remains a forecast of possible or probable outcome only.

Prognosis can change with time, with the progress of healing, the development of complications, the effects of treatment, even with a change of diagnosis. Any given prognosis should carry that rider. The unexpected can always happen, and Murphy's Law is always with us. Further injury may alter behaviour, particularly if the original injury has left an impairment. An impaired structure can be vulnerable to further injury and that injury may come out of the physical and psychological stresses of work and daily living. Age may modify the end result. There may be continuing deterioration. If there is residual impairment, deterioration may be delayed in onset. An example of this is the osteoarthrosis that can follow injury to a joint. There are four possible outcomes to such a complication (Smith, 1986).

1. The joint is left so destroyed as to result in immediate disability and handicap. The condition may then remain static or deteriorate. Increasing disability can increase handicap, or paradoxically, decrease it. An example is the stiff subtalar joint after a fracture of the calcaneus. A painful fibrous ankylosis imposing a severe handicap may become a painless ankylosis, possibly by surgical fusion. Complete absence of subtalar movement amounts to a greater disability but the abolition of pain will diminish the handicap.
2. There may be no impairment at the end of treatment but degenerative changes can develop later causing disability and handicap.
3. There may be residual impairment which constitutes no disability at the time but leads to progressive disability.
4. There may be residual impairment producing a degree of disability which inflicts no handicap and which never progresses.

When receiving a prognosis in a medical report, the lawyer will wish to know the following:

1. The prognosis at that time, concerning the nature, risks, duration and cost of any further treatment.
2. Whether work is possible in that period.
3. What will be the precise impairment or disability at the end of treatment?
4. Will a return to the pre-accident occupation be possible?
5. Will the patient be able to continue at that occupation until normal retiring age?

6. If not, what alternative employment would be appropriate?
7. Will the patient be at a disadvantage applying for alternative employment on the open labour market?
8. Will leisure activities be affected?
9. If there is permanent disability, will there be a need for the provision of continuing care?
10. Will there be delayed complications? If so when? What effect will they have on the above?
11. Has the expectancy of life changed?

Some of these questions will be unanswerable. If they are, the reporting surgeon should say so unequivocally, and should not make 'guesstimates' which may later prove to be misleading.

An opinion as to outcome may be expressed in terms of possibilities or probabilities. A rough rule is that 'possible' describes an outcome with a smaller than 50% chance of occurring, 'probable' one with a greater than 50% chance. The phrase 'on balance of probabilities' allows an opinion to be given with authority, yet with the understanding that the unforeseen may modify the forecast.

Multiple injuries and the systemic effects of injury

In this book, individual injuries are dealt with in sequence. In high-velocity injuries, multiple injuries are the rule rather than the exception. Visceral injuries can be life threatening and their management takes priority in the immediate post-traumatic period. They are usually resolved quickly, one way or the other, and residual impairment and disability is the result of the musculoskeletal injury. Multiple fractures may delay recovery and make greater demand on rehabilitation services than isolated injuries; but they do not, as a rule, adversely affect prognosis except in special anatomical circumstances. Fractures above and below a joint may produce more residual impairment of that joint's function than a single adjacent fracture. A nerve injury complicating a joint injury may so delay the return of movement to that joint as to result in permanent impairment. A minor fracture, undetected amongst other major lesions, may emerge as the sole cause of residual disability.

The systemic effects of injury, in particular blood loss, can also be threatening to life. Other complications include venous thrombosis and embolus, fat embolism, traumatic renal ischaemia and infection. Each can cause residual impairment and therefore have an effect on prognosis.

The association of injury with the onset of, or the recognition of, disease is contentious. The obvious example in musculoskeletal injury is osteoarthrosis, which as been discussed above. Other systemic diseases, such as rheumatoid arthritis, may appear to have been triggered by the accident. It is wise to obtain the opinion of a physician with special knowledge of the condition when the question does arise.

Pathological fractures provide a special instance of how injury can precipitate recognition of underlying disease.

Some lesions of bone so destroy its integrity as to cause spontaneous fracture, that is a fracture which occurs without external force being applied. Others weaken bone structure so that a fracture occurs following a physical force which would not break normal bone. This force may be minimal and, applied to a bone affected by a lesion which would inevitably progress to spontaneous fracture, merely accelerates the inevitable. Sometimes the fracture may be held to be beneficial in that it induces healing of the defect. Even in undiagnosed malignant disease, a pathological fracture may permit recognition of the lesion, treatment and possibly an enhanced expectation of life.

The prognosis is obviously that of the underlying disease, but treatment may modify its subsequent natural history.

The psychological effects of injury and their effect on prognosis

Physical injury is accompanied by emotional stress. This can have metabolic effects immediately after the accident, but the healing of fractures is dependent on local vascular and systemic biochemical factors. Residual disability, however, is significantly influenced by non-physical circumstances, as is the speed with which recovery occurs. This effect, paradoxically, is seen more often in injuries which do not produce identifiable structural lesions. The psychological factors influencing the speed of recovery and residual handicap are diverse. They include occupational, social and domestic influences.

Self-employed people return to work quicker than those in paid employment. Injuries sustained at work take longer to heal than those not sustained at work, and have a higher incidence of disability. To interpret these facts as meaning that people injured at work deliberately prolong their recovery and exaggerate their residual symptoms is naive. The issues are more complex and require understanding if terms like 'malingering,' 'functional overlay' or 'low pain threshold' are not to be loosely used in medical reports.

The facts are available. Reviews consistently show that patients injured at work (and the injury may be no more than the accepted physical stresses of a given occupation) take longer to return to work than if they are injured outside working hours (Leavitt, Garron and McNeil, 1982; Sander and Meyer, 1986).

Faced with a patient whose symptoms are not adequately explained by his signs, in other words, whose subjective impairment is disproportionate to his structural impairment, the surgeon must decide whether the patient is simply exaggerating his symptoms, suffering from compensation neurosis or malingering (Woodyard, 1982). Woodyard feels that patients affected by compensation neurosis have an excellent prognosis, but other authorities do not agree and suggest that psychiatric treatment and assessment are necessary (Ellard, 1970; Hodge, 1971). The orthopaedic surgeon is advised to record his observations, to avoid labelling a patient as a malingerer unless he has seen him carry out an action which he claimed he could not perform, and to be guarded in his prognosis.

References

American Medical Association (1977) *Guides to the Evaluation of Permanent Impairment,* American Medical Association, Chicago

Ellard, J. (1970) Psychological reactions to compensable injury. *Medical Journal of Australia,* **2**, 349–355

Hodge, J. R. (1971) The whiplash neurosis. *Psychosomatics,* **12**, 245–249

Leavitt, F., Garron, D. C. and McNeil, T. W. (1982) Organic status, psychological disturbance and pain characteristics in low back pain patients on compensation. *Spine,* **7**, 398–424

Sander, R. A. and Meyer, J. E. (1986) Relation of disability to compensation in railway workers. *Spine,* **11**, 141–143

Smith, D. H. (1986) *Medical Reports on Compensation Claimants,* University of Edinburgh, Edinburgh

World Health Organisation (1986) *International Classification of Impairments, Disabilities and Handicaps,* Geneva

Woodyard, J. E. (1982) Diagnosis and prognosis in compensation claims. *Annals of the Royal College of Surgeons,* **4**, 191–194

Part 1

The spine and pelvis

1

Injuries of the thoracolumbar spine

The disability produced by transection of the spinal cord is total and devastating. The resulting handicap can be reduced by skilled care and rehabilitation, to the point where a return to useful life in the community can be achieved. The disability is permanent. Continuing care and support is necessary. Prognosis in these depressing injuries is best made by experts in spinal cord injury, and not by orthopaedic surgeons who do not have a clinical attachment to a spinal injuries centre.

Not all injuries of the bony vertebral column or its accessory structures are associated with spinal cord, or cauda equina lesions. Their management occurs in general hospitals, by orthopaedic surgeons. This section is concerned with such lesions.

In no area of injury can prognosis be more difficult or contentious than in the lower back. Some injuries are clearly identifiable and then the picture is clearer, but others are difficult to diagnose; they may be associated with pre-existing degenerative change which may or may not have been productive of symptoms. Assessment is made more complicated by the fact that radiographic appearances, more often than not, bear little or no relation to the severity or natural history of these conditions.

Bony injury of the thoracolumbar spine

Burst fractures, fracture dislocations and translocations of the vertebrae which have not caused cord damage are unstable and dangerous. Their immediate prognosis depends on the success or failure of management to maintain stability. When stability has been assured, the functional end result is comparable to that following stable fractures of the vertebral bodies.

Compression fractures of thoracic or lumbar vertebral bodies

These are stable fractures which unite readily leaving little clinical deformity, but which have a deserved reputation for causing long-term problems. Some reviews, dealing with short-term results in service personnel, are optimistic (Watson-Jones, 1955). One large Australian series, with an average 9-year follow up of 216 patients, found that while residual symptoms were common, no patient required operative treatment for relief of pain. There was no correlation between the severity of symptoms and radiographic findings such as spontaneous fusion, loss of vertebral height, persistent kyphosis or encroachment into the spinal canal (Taylor *et al.*, 1986). Others paint a gloomier picture. Another Australian paper, contemporary with the above, found a 'high incidence' of chronic pain and disability in 82 patients (Osti, Frazer and Cornish, 1986). In a review of 152 injured Nottinghamshire coal miners, 60% had residual low back pain (Nicoll, 1949). Of Nicoll's patients, 88% returned to work, but only half of these returned to work at the coal face. The remainder were found light work either underground or on the surface, and 'light work' in the British Coal Industry means just that. Nicoll also found little correlation between radiographic appearance and residual disability. He commented on the greater frequency of residual low back pain against pain felt at the site of the fracture and concluded that this was due to soft tissue scarring from gravitational haematoma (Nicoll, 1949).

Young's review of 623 Canadian patients found that 75% experienced continuing pain, with 25% of these incapacitated from work. Again, he found no correlation between radiographic appearances and clinical findings (Young, 1973). However, one paper, while recording a comparable incidence of residual symptoms, states that severe radiographic changes were associated with severe pain (Day and Kokan, 1977).

References

Day, B. and Kokan, D. (1977) Compression fractures of the thoracic and lumbar spine from compensable injuries. *Clinical Orthopaedics,* **124**, 173–176

Nicoll, E. A. (1949) Fractures of the dorso-lumbar spine. *Journal of Bone and Joint Surgery,* **31B**, 376–394

Osti, O., Frazer, R. D. and Cornish, B. L. (1986) Fractures and fracture dislocations in the lumbar spine. *Journal of Bone and Joint Surgery,* **68B**, 334

Taylor, T. K. F., Ruff, S. J., Alglietti, P. L., Dimuria, G. V., Marcucci, M. and Novembri, A. (1986) Long term results of wedge fractures of dorso-lumbar spine. *Journal of Bone and Joint Surgery,* **68B**, 334

Watson-Jones, R. (1955) *Fractures and Joint Injuries*, 4th edn, Vol. II, E. & S. Livingstone, Edinburgh and London, p. 960

Young, M. H. (1973) Long term consequences of stable fractures of the thoracic and lumbar vertebral bodies. *Journal of Bone and Joint Surgery,* **55B**, 295–300

Table 1.1

Injury	Stable compression fractures of thoracic and lumbar vertebral bodies	
Structural impairment	Deformity of vertebral body Loss of vertebral height Persistent kyphosis Spontaneous fusion	Radiographic appearances not correlated with clinical result
Subjective impairment	Pain 1. at site of fracture 2. low back pain Stiffness, does not result in appreciable disability Muscle weakness	In up to 75–80%
Disability and handicap	Incapacity to work – 12–25% Incapacity for heavy physical work – up to 40%	
Comments	Views differ on the value of intensive rehabilitation programmes Watson-Jones and Nicoll were in favour, but Young found that the worst results were in those who had spent longest in rehabilitation centres. He felt that residual disability could be assessed early. All reviews are long term and the results were not influenced by compensation claims	

Isthmic spondylolisthesis

The defect in the pars interarticularis is accepted as being an impact or fatigue fracture (Murray and Colwill, 1968; Wiltse, Newman and MacNab, 1976; Cyron, Hutton and Troup, 1976). The presence of the defect is not necessarily associated with symptoms, but displacement is (Nachemson, 1976). The degree of slip equates with the severity of the clinical picture, and it is important in management to know whether further displacement will occur. In adults it is extremely unlikely. In children and adolescents there is a 15% risk of further slip (Blackburne and Velikas, 1977). They found the following to be predisposing factors.

1. The ratio of male to female in progressive slipping was 7 : 5; in the whole series it was 69 : 73.
2. The risk increases during the adolescent growth spurt.
3. A slip of less than one-third diameter is unlikely to further slip beyond one-third. A slip of over one-third diameter when first seen may progress to total diameter displacement.
4. The presence of a midline lumbosacral defect and other vertebral anomalies increases the likelihood of further displacement.

References

Blackburne, J. S. and Velikas, E. P. (1977) Spondylolisthesis in children and adolescents. *Journal of Bone and Joint Surgery,* **59B**, 490–494

Cyron, B. M., Hutton, W. R. and Troup, J. D. G. (1976) Spondylolytic fractures. *Journal of Bone and Joint Surgery,* **58B**, 462–470

Murray, R. O. and Colwill, M. R. (1968) Stress fractures of the pars interarticularis. *Proceedings of the Royal Society of Medicine,* **61**, 555–557

Nachemson, A. L. (1976) The lumbar spine. *Spine,* **1**, 59–71

Wiltse, L. L., Newman, P. H. and Macnab, I. (1976) Classification of spondylolysis and spondylolisthesis. *Clinical Orthopaedics and Related Research,* **17**, 23–29

Compression vertebral body fractures in postmenopausal osteoporosis

These are pathological fractures produced by trivial violence or occurring spontaneously in osteoporotic bone. When the fracture occurs there has already been considerable loss of bone mass. Severe pain settles within 6–8 weeks but the risk of further fracture is high. There is little evidence that treatment, other than the encouragement of physical exercise, has any prophylactic value. Risk features have been identified (Buchanan *et al.*, 1987) as:

1. A slender build.
2. A sedentary life style.
3. Deficiency of calcium.
4. Smoking.
5. Excess alcohol intake.
6. Deficiency of oestrogen.

Reference

Buchanan, J. R., Myers, C., Greer, R. B., Lloyd, T. and Varano, L. A. (1987) Assessment of the risk of vertebral fracture in menopausal women. *Journal of Bone and Joint Surgery,* **69A**, 212–218

Lesions of the lumbar intervertebral disc

The short-term results of surgical excision of prolapsed intervertebral discs are excellent. Long-term follow up reveals some deterioration with time, but overall the results are good. An Oswestry review of 102 patients showed that 82% had excellent long-term (5–11 years) results, with 65% of patients returning to heavy work. However, 17% had no relief of pain. Poor results were apparent within 2 years and were unlikely to appear thereafter (Chabra and Eiseinstein, 1989). Equally good results in terms of relief of radicular pain were given by Hanley and Shapiro (1989), but they found that 14% of their cases developed disabling low back pain. This symptom correlated with the patient's age (those over 40 doing worse), heavy smoking and an injury sustained at work. A great many papers have been written on the results of surgical discectomy giving broadly similar results, and I have been selective. One controlled prospective study of 126 patients randomized into operative and non-operative treatment showed that while the results at 1 year were considerably better after operation than non-operative management, 4 and 10 years later there was no difference in the results (Weber, 1983).

The behaviour of the prolapsed disc in the adolescent is different. Neurological signs are scarce and recovery after operation is prolonged, up to 8 months in some cases (Bolus, 1973). Nevertheless, many reports describe excellent results after disc excision (Bolus, 1973; Grobelaar, Simmons and Barrington, 1979; Taylor, 1982). The Oswestry experience is more pessimistic. Of 21 adolescents treated by discectomy, eleven did well, four only fair and six had poor results (Curtin, O'Brien and Park, 1977).

References

Bolus, S. (1973) Herniated intervertebral lumbar disc in the teenager. *Journal of Bone and Joint Surgery,* **55B**, 273–278

Chabra, M. and Eiseinstein, S. (1989) The natural history after lumbar intervertebral discectomy. *The Oswestrian,* **1**, 1–6

Curtin, J., O'Brien, J. P. and Park, W. P. (1977) Natural history of surgically treated herniated lumbar intervertebral disc in the adolescent. *Journal of Bone and Joint Surgery,* **59B**, 506

Grobelaar, L. J., Simmons, E. H. and Barrington, T. W. (1979) Intervertebral disc herniation in the adolescent. *Journal of Bone and Joint Surgery,* **61B**, 256

Hanley, E. N. and Shapiro, D. E. (1989) The development of low back pain after excision of a lumbar disc. *Journal of Bone and Joint Surgery,* **71A**, 719–721

Taylor, T. K. F. (1982) Lumbar intervertebral disc lesion in children and adolescents. *Journal of Bone and Joint Surgery,* **64B**, 135

Weber, H. (1983) Lumbar disc herniation. *Spine,* **8**, 131–140

Low back pain without bony injury

The chronic low back pain syndrome after industrial injury is common, as is the chronic low back pain syndrome after occupational stress, leisure injury or without any injury at all. Attempts have been made to break down the syndrome into diagnostic classifications. Some causes of pain can be identified clinically, by standard or contrast radiography or by the newer methods of imaging. They include the traumatic lesions of spondylolysis and spondylolisthesis, prolapsed intervertebral discs, tears of the annulus fibrosus, spinal stenosis, ankylosing spondylitis and others (White, Derby and Wynne, 1980). Increasingly sophisticated methods of imaging will decrease the number of patients whose pain source cannot be identified, as will better understanding of natural history (Fairbank *et al.*, 1981; Yang and King, 1984; Eiseinstein and Parry, 1987). There remain, and will probably always remain, patients whose lesion is unknown and whose response to treatment is disappointing.

Prognosis in these patients is a depressing exercise and beset with conflict over the comparative contribution of physical and psychological factors to the disability. Statistical reviews are gloomy (Beals and Hickman, 1972; Frymoyer *et al.*, 1980).

Certain points in individual prognosis need to be emphasized. There is no correlation between the plain radiographic appearances of the lumbar spine and the severity of the clinical condition. Many radiographic appearances are of no value at all in determining the cause of low back pain or in predicting which individual is at risk (Frymoyer *et al.*, 1984). It is doubtful whether changes such as spondylolysis, retrolisthesis or scoliosis are relevant. Nachemson (1976) identifies the following as definitely significant: spondylolisthesis; Scheurmann's disease; congenital or traumatic kyphosis; marked multiple disc space narrowing; ankylosing spondylitis. Other authorities add the appearance of traction spurs as being indicative of lumbar instability and hence relevant to the clinical picture (MacNab, 1971).

All of these radiographic changes can, of course, be seen in individuals who have never experienced significant back pain in their working lives.

Assessment in the individual case must therefore be made on clinical grounds. Unfortunately, physical signs or their absence can be interpreted differently by different examiners. The adversarial nature of civil actions for damages in British courts means that each litigant is examined on behalf of opposing sides; and lawyers tend to choose as examiners those whom they know take either a jaundiced or a benevolent view of human motives. Completely opposite interpretations of physical signs result and the case is usually resolved by a compromise between those views, by lay, that is judicial, adjudication between the two.

Pain cannot be measured. Back stiffness from pain can be influenced by a multitude of factors. Patients with chronic back problems have good days and bad days and their physical signs will vary from time to time.

Waddell *et al.* (1980) have drawn attention to what they call non-organic physical signs in low back pain, that is to say, physical signs which cannot be explained on the basis of any known structural lesion in the spine. These have been familiar to discerning clinicians for a long time. They include obvious over-reactions such as disproportionate descriptions of the severity of the pain and exaggerated responses to examination such as dramatic collapses, grimaces, groaning when carrying out simple manoeuvres, contraction of antagonistic muscles and widespread tenderness to light touch or deep pressure. The wise clinician, however, will be careful in his interpretation of these findings. A patient being examined for a medical report by the 'other side' is more apprehensive than he is in a routine consultation. Cultural mores may impose a varying degree of stoicism. Some patients genuinely believe that their doctor will not think they have a serious complaint unless their pain is described as agony.

More reliable indications of non-organic disease are found in what Waddell calls simulation and distraction signs. Simulation signs include low back pain felt when pressure is applied to the standing patient's head, or low back pain produced when the shoulders and pelvis are passively rotated together. The well-known distraction sign is that of restricted straight leg raising in the prone patient with full straight leg raising in the same patient sitting upright or with his legs dangling over the side of the couch. 'Stocking' anaesthesia and motor paralysis in the presence of normal muscle tone suggest hysteria rather than functional overlay (Waddell *et al.*, 1980).

Unfortunately, these non-organic signs are only valuable if the patient is not aware of them. If they are itemized in the report, and if the patient sees that report, they will not be present again.

The patient's history since the accident is probably the single most helpful feature in prognosis. It has been shown that the period of incapacity, as measured by time away from work, is four times longer when the injury is sustained at work than when it is not (Sander and Meyers, 1986). The longer a patient is away from work the less likely he is to return to his pre-accident occupation.

Prognosis in patients with a chronic disability must cover those tasks and occupations which may or may not be within the individual's capacity. His or her specific handicap must be identified. This is largely self-evident as the patient can identify those specific movements and manoeuvres which aggravate his symptoms. Some physically demanding work involving bending, lifting and carrying is readily understood as being prohibitive for chronic low back pain patients. It is now recognized that occupations involving dynamic loading and the vibration of multiple impacts, such as truck driving, are unsuitable for low back pain patients (Frymoyer *et al.*, 1980; Wilder *et al.*, 1982; Sandover, 1983).

An interesting review (Pederson, 1981) has come from a general practice in Denmark, identifying prognostic features in patients consulting their family doctor. The review does not differentiate between those giving a history of injury and those not, except to observe that the onset of pain while at work, without specific injury, results in a greater period of unfitness to work. Other features indicating a long or relapsing course were:

1. More than three previous episodes of low back pain.
2. Gradual onset of symptoms.
3. Pain referred distal to the knee.
4. More than 4 weeks delay in reporting symptoms.

By implication this shows a poorer prognosis in patients who did not experience a definite episode of injury.

References

Beals, R. K. and Hickman, N. E. (1972) Industrial injuries of the low back. *Journal of Bone and Joint Surgery,* **54A**, 1593–1611

Eiseinstein, S. M. and Parry, C. R. (1987) The lumbar facet arthrosis syndrome. *Journal of Bone and Joint Surgery,* **69B**, 3–7

Fairbank, J. C., Park, W. M., McCall, I. W. and O'Brien, J. P. (1981) Apophyseal injection in primary low back pain syndromes. *Spine,* **6**, 598–605

Frymoyer, J. W., Newberg, A., Pope, M. H., Wilder, D. G., Clements, J. and McPherson, B. (1984) Spine radiographs in patients with low back pain. *Journal of Bone and Joint Surgery,* **66A**, 1049–1053

Frymoyer, J. W., Pope, M. H., Costanza, M. C., Rosen, J. C., Coggin, J. E. and Wilder, D. G. (1980) Epidemiological studies of low back pain. *Spine,* **5**, 419–423

McNab, I. (1971) The traction spur. *Journal of Bone and Joint Surgery,* **53A**, 663–670

Nachemson, A. L. (1976) The lumbar spine. *Spine,* **1**, 59–71

Pederson, J. (1981) Prognostic indicators in low back pain. *Journal of the Royal College of General Practitioners,* **31**, 209–216

Sander, R. A. and Meyers, J. E. (1986) Relation of disability to compensation in railway workers. *Spine,* **11**, 141–143

Sandover, J. (1983) Dynamic loading as a source of low back pain. *Spine,* **8**, 653–657

Waddell, G., McCullough, J. A., Kummel, E. and Venner, R. M. (1980) Non-organic physical signs in low back pain. *Spine,* **5**, 117–128

White, A. R., Derby, R. and Wynne, G. (1980) A diagnostic classification of low back pain. *Spine,* **5**, 83–86

Wilder, D. G., Woodworth, B. B., Frymoyer, J. W. and Pope, M. H. (1982) Vibration and the human spine. *Spine,* **7**, 243–254

Yang, K. H. and King, A. I. (1984) Mechanism of facet load transmission as a hypothesis for low back pain. *Spine,* **9**, 557–565

2

Fractures of the cervical spine

Fractures and fracture dislocations of the cervical spine which have been reduced and are not associated with neurological damage do well. The prognosis depends on the stability of the reduced fracture or dislocation. Stability of the cervical spine depends on the integrity of the supporting structures; bilateral facet dislocation, for example, can only occur if there has been complete disruption of the posterior ligamentous complex. The decision to fuse the reduced dislocation lies in the province of management, but 10% of reduced and unfused cervical fracture dislocations remain unstable after the anticipated period of healing has passed (White, Southwick and Panjabi, 1976; McSweeney, 1980). Methods of forecasting instability have been described by White and his co-authors.

Some features are potentially unstable even although signs of instability are not immediately apparent on first presentation. They have been termed 'hidden flexion injuries' (Webb *et al.*, 1976) and are recognized by the radiographic appearances of:

1. Widening of the interspinous space.
2. Intervertebral subluxation.
3. Loss or lordosis.

Simple compression fractures of cervical vertebrae are, on the whole, stable but judgement should be reserved. Mazur and Stauffer (1983) reported a series of 27 cases of simple compression fractures of cervical vertebrae, treated by orthotic splintage. Of these, 21 healed and the patients became, and remained, symptom-free during a 30-month follow up. However, six developed persistent pain, and radiographs 12 weeks after injury showed abnormal movement. None of the six fulfilled any of Webb's or White's criteria for instability. Prognosis in such injuries must be guarded until sufficient time, probably at least 6 months, has elapsed to be sure that residual instability is not present.

Delayed union and non-union of cervical spine fractures are rare, and confined to the level above C.2.

Fractures of the odontoid are classified according to their level. Type I fractures occur through the apex of the process, Type II through the waist and Type III extend into the body of the axis. Non-union occurs in 36% of Type II lesions. Untreated, this can result in atlanto-axial instability with the ever present danger of spinal cord compromise.

Traumatic atlanto-axial instability in the presence of an intact odontoid process can only occur if the transverse arm of the cruciate ligament has been ruptured. As the ligament is a stronger structure than the dens itself this lesion should not occur in the healthy spine (Werne, 1957). Cases have been reported, however, in children and adults (Highland and Aronson, 1986; De Beer *et al.*, 1988). The ruptured ligament will not heal and these injuries are unstable.

Atlanto-occipital displacement should not be compatible with life, but some patients have survived with an unstable atlanto-occipital subluxation. They are at considerable risk if the lesion is not recognized and stabilized.

Malunion of cervical fractures is common. They do not, as a rule, give rise to any problems. Movement of the neck is not restricted to a degree apparent to the patient. There may be compromise of nerve roots, from compression in the vertebral foramina or from irritation of posterior roots adjacent to osteoarthrotic apophyseal joints (McSweeney, 1980).

Radiographic appearances of degeneration appear adjacent to fractured segments. It is reasonable to hold that the appearance of these changes has been accelerated by the injury, but, as such changes are universal with normal ageing, it is not possible to express such acceleration in mathematical terms. In any event the appearances on X-ray do not correlate with any symptoms experienced or signs exhibited by the patient.

References

De Beer, J. D. V., Thomas, M., Walters, J. and Anderson, P. (1988) Traumatic atlanto-axial subluxation. *Journal of Bone and Joint Surgery,* **70B**, 652–656

Highland, T. R. and Aronson, D. D. (1986) Traumatic rupture of cervical transverse ligament with normal odontoid. *Spine,* **11**, 73–75

Mazur, J. M. and Stauffer, S. E. (1983) Unrecognized instability with simple cervical compression fractures. *Spine,* **8**, 687–692

McSweeney, T. (1980) Fractures and fracture dislocations of the cervical spine. In *Disorders of the Cervical Spine* (ed. T. E. Jeffreys), Butterworths, London, pp. 48–80

Webb, J. K., Broughton, B. K., McSweeney, T. and Park, W. M. (1976) Hidden flexion injury of cervical spine. *Journal of Bone and Joint Surgery,* **58B**, 322–327
Werne, S. (1957) Studies in spontaneous atlas dislocation. *Acta Orthopaedica Scandinavia Supplement* XXII
White, A. A., Southwick, W. O. and Panjabi, M. M. (1976) Clinical instability in the lower cervical spine. *Spine,* **1**, 15–27

3

Soft tissue injuries of the cervical spine

Extension-acceleration injuries of the neck are called 'whiplash' injuries by lawyers, patients and, regrettably, by doctors. I have objected to this catachresis (Jeffreys, 1980), as has its originator (Crowe, 1928), but the term remains popular. In my opinion it is an emotive expression, and using it adversely affects prognosis.

It has been known for a long time that a substantial number of these patients do badly, with up to 45% experiencing residual symptoms 5 years after injury, and over 2 years after litigation has been resolved (McNab, 1964; Hohl, 1974). These earlier reports were written before seat belts and head restraints became standard equipment in motor cars, and one would have hoped that their introduction had reduced the frequency and severity of these injuries. That does not seem to have happened (Greenfield and Ilfield, 1977; Deans *et al.*, 1987).

Attempts have been made to identify clinical or radiographic features in the recently injured patient, which can assist in prognosis. Hohl's seminal paper describes pain or numbness radiating into the arms as significant in predicting a long duration of symptoms, but felt that the presence or absence of abnormal physical signs at first examination were not significant. In his series, age was of no consequence but women tended to recover more slowly than men (Hohl, 1964). Greenfield and Ilfield (1977) also found that the patient's age had no effect on the final outcome, but that the symptom of pain radiating between the shoulder blades was the only finding consistent with a poor prognosis.

The radiographic signs have been assessed. Greenfield and Ilfield (1977) found that loss of the normal lordotic curve bore no relation to the time to recovery, but Hohl (1964) wrote that a break in lordosis at one segment was significant. Norris and Watt (1983) assessed 61 cases within 7 days of injury and divided them into three clinical groups: those with symptoms but no signs, those with symptoms and a stiff neck and those with neurological signs. Of the eight patients in the last group, six were no better or worse after their litigation had been settled. They found a higher incidence of radiographic abnormality in this third group, and felt that alteration of the cervical curve was associated with a poor result. Perhaps more importantly, they found that 40% of their third group showed pre-existing degenerative change on the neck radiographs, against 26% in their first group (Norris and Watt, 1983).

Despite documented evidence that there is little correlation between radiographic degeneration and clinical presentation, lawyers wish to know whether neck injuries will result in the development, or the accelerated development, of degenerative joint or intervertebral disc disease. With age of course these changes become universal, and the incidence accelerates with age. Whereas 16% of people between 30 and 40 years old show radiographic degeneration, this incidence rises to 25% between 40 and 50 years of age (Freidenberg and Miller, 1963). Hohl (1964) found that 39% of his patients developed radiographic changes during his follow up period of a minimal 5 years after injury. This is more than would be expected from normal ageing, but he did not find correlation between radiographic change and residual symptoms.

Accepting that symptoms can persist for over 5 years in up to 45% of people so injured, it remains to be considered what effect litigation itself has on continuing symptoms. McNab (1964) was in no doubt that it had no effect. Other authors have not been so sure (Breck and Van Norman, 1971; Jeffreys, 1980). Norris and Watt (1983) found that all of their third group pursued litigation while only half of their first group did. Breck and Van Norman (1971) found that the duration of treatment in litigants was four times as prolonged as in non-litigants, and Hohl (1964) reported that 83% of those whose claim had been settled within 6 months of the accident were symptom-free at his review against 38% of those whose lawsuits had dragged out more than 18 months.

Norris and Watt (1983) felt that those patients injured in a stationary vehicle did worse; and Grundy has pointed out that the stationary victim of a rear end impact is, that rarity in road accidents, totally blameless in the eyes of the law. Grundy's long-term review paints the most pessimistic picture of all, with 62% of patients still having symptoms at least 10 years after injury. Of these, 44% had not returned to their pre-accident occupation, and 62.5% had been forced to modify their leisure activities (Hodgson and Grundy, 1989).

Flexion and lateral flexion acceleration injuries do far better. The original force is less severe than in extension-acceleration and the distribution of responsibility for the accident is less well established.

References

Breck, L. W. and Van Norman, R. W. (1971) Medicolegal aspects of cervical sprains. *Clinical Orthopaedics,* **74**, 124–128

Crowe, H. E. (1928) Injuries to the cervical spine. Annual Meeting, Western Orthopaedic Association

Deans, G. T., Magalliard, J. N., Kerr, M. and Rutherford, W. H. (1987) Neck sprain. *Injury,* **18**, 10–12

Freidenberg, Z. B. and Miller, W. I. (1963) Degenerative disc disease of the cervical spine. *Journal of Bone and Joint Surgery,* **45A**, 1171–1178

Greenfield, J. and Ilfield, F. W. (1977) Acute cervical strain. *Clinical Orthopaedics,* **122**, 196–200

Hodgson, S. P. and Grundy, M. (1989) Whiplash injuries: their long term prognosis and its relationship to compensation. *Neuro-orthopaedics,* **7**, 88–91

Hohl, M. (1974) Soft tissue injuries of the neck in automobile accidents. *Journal of Bone and Joint Surgery,* **56A**, 1675–1682

Jeffreys, T. E. (1980) *Disorders of the Cervical Spine*, Butterworths, London

McNab, I. (1964) Acceleration injuries of the cervical spine. *Journal of Bone and Joint Surgery,* **46A**, 1797–1799

Norris, S. H. and Watt, I. (1983) The prognosis of neck injuries resulting from rear end vehicle collisions. *Journal of Bone and Joint Surgery,* **65B**, 608–611

Table 3.1

Injury	extension-acceleration injuries of the cervical spine
Structural impairment	Soft tissue injury to anterior supporting structures of neck Vertebral artery compromise Sympathetic impairment Horizontal tear of intervertebral disc
Subjective impairment	Neck pain and stiffness Pain/numbness in arms or interscapular area Headaches Vertigo, dizziness, dysphagia, blurred vision } Symptoms persist in 45% up to 5 years, 10% up to 10 years
Disability and handicap	10% forced to change their occupation, or modify their leisure activities
Comments	Features suggesting a poor prognosis when first seen are: 1. Restricted neck movement 2. Interscapular pain 3. Neurological signs of root involvement 4. Degenerative change on standard X-ray films

4 Fractures of the pelvis

The detailed classifications of pelvic fractures that have been proposed in recent years reflect the tendency towards operative stabilization of these injuries (Pennal *et al.*, 1980; Tile, 1988). Prognosis for medical reports can be covered by the simpler grouping used by Watson-Jones (1955): (1) avulsion fractures; (2) fractures and dislocations of the pelvic ring; (3) fractures of the sacrum and coccyx.

Avulsion fractures

Caused by muscular violence these fractures are seen at the anterior superior and inferior iliac spines, and the ischial tuberosity. Some degree of malunion is usual but residual disability is absent or minimal in the majority of patients.

Fractures and dislocations of the pelvic ring

Undisplaced fractures of the pubic rami are common injuries in the elderly. They occur through osteoporotic bone, with minimal violence. Union occurs within a few weeks and there is no residual disability. In the young patient symptoms tend to be more severe and low back pain is common. Union is almost invariable without functional impairment although non-union has been reported (Dunn and Morris, 1968).

Separation of the pubic rami must be accompanied by a corresponding separation elsewhere in the pelvic ring. Separation of the symphysis of less than one inch leaves no residual disability although pain and local tenderness may persist for 2 years or more after injury (Holdsworth, 1948).

Severe disruptions of the pelvic ring are responsible for prolonged morbidity and a significant incidence of residual disability. The residual problems are associated with shortening from vertical displacement of the hemipelvis, and sacro-iliac joint injury. Low back pain is a residual symptom in over half of patients (Holdsworth, 1948; Dunn and Morris, 1968; Slatis and Huittenen, 1972). In Holdsworth's series less than half his patients with sacro-iliac joint disruption were able to return to their pre-accident occupation.

Major fractures of the pelvis can be associated with injury to blood vessels, nerves and pelvic viscera, in particular the bladder and urethra. Neurological lesions do badly; incomplete recovery is the rule (Huittenen and Slatis, 1971).

Rupture of the urethra can be followed by incontinence, stricture and impotence. Permanent impotence occurs in nearly half of patients with urethral rupture (Chambers and Balfour, 1963).

Fractures of the sacrum and coccyx

Isolated crack fractures of the sacrum are seen from time to time. They unite quickly. Separated fractures more often accompany other pelvic fractures and the incidence of reported complications are high. Malunion, non-union, permanent neurological defects and persistent low back pain have been reported (Hazlett, 1980; Foy, 1988).

Injuries of the coccyx include contusion, fracture and dislocation. Coccygeal pain is notoriously slow to resolve, persisting for 12–18 months after injury. Symptoms persisting for longer should raise the suspicion of a central disc prolapse at the lumbosacral level (H. J. Richards, 1960, personal communication).

References

Chambers, H. L. and Balfour, J. (1963) The incidence of impotence following pelvic fractures with associated urinary tract injury. *Journal of Urology*, **89**, 702–703

Dunn, A. W. and Morris, H. D. (1968) Fractures and dislocations of the pelvis. *Journal of Bone and Joint Surgery*, **50A**, 1639–1648

Foy, M. A. (1988) Morbidity following isolated fractures of the sacrum. *Injury*, **19**, 379–380

Hazlett, J. W. (1980) Fractures of the sacrum. *Journal of Bone and Joint Surgery*, **62B**, 130–131

Holdsworth, F. W. (1948) Dislocation and fracture dislocation of the pelvis. *Journal of Bone and Joint Surgery*, **30B**, 461–466

Huittenen, V. M. and Slatis, P. (1971) Nerve injury in double vertical pelvic fractures. *Acta Chirurgica Scandinavia,* **138**, 571–575

Pennal, G. F., Tile, M., Waddell, J. P. and Garside, H. (1980) Pelvic disruption; assessment and classification. *Clinical Orthopaedics,* **151**, 12–21

Slatis, P. and Huittenen, V. M. (1972) Double vertical fractures of the pelvis. *Acta Chirurgica Scandinavia,* **138**, 799–807

Tile, M. (1988) Pelvic ring fractures: should they be fixed? *Journal of Bone and Joint Surgery,* **70B**, 1–2

Watson-Jones, R. (1955) *Fractures and Joint Injuries*, 4th edn, Vol. II, E. & S. Livingstone, Edinburgh and London, pp. 934–945

Table 4.1

Injury	Fractures of the pelvis and disruptions of pelvic ring
Structural impairment	Malunion. Shortening. Sacro-iliac subluxation. Pelvic obliquity. Non-union 3%
Subjective impairment	Low back pain. 50–60% complain of persistent pain. Limp
Disability and handicap	50% unable to return to pre-accident occupation
Comments	Morbidity is prolonged. Rehabilitation may continue for over 1 year

Table 4.2

Injury	Fractures of the pelvis, visceral complications
Structural impairment	Arterial injury Neurological injury – lower lumbar and sacral roots. Recovery always incomplete Genito-urinary injury – bladder rupture – urethral rupture leading to stricture, incontinence – impotence
Subjective impairment	Residual motor or sensory loss of varying degree
Disability and handicap	Impotence permanent in 50%. Prognosis worsens with age
Comments	Delay prognosis in neurological lesions (including impotence) for 12–18 months to allow full potential for recovery

Table 4.3

Injury	Coccydynia
Structural impairment	1. Contusion, Fracture, Dislocation } of coccyx 2. Central prolapse of lumbosacral disc
Subjective impairment	Pain on sitting and exertion
Disability and handicap	Those whose occupations involve prolonged sitting are handicapped
Comments	Recovery is prolonged and, in some, symptoms persist indefinitely

Part 2

The upper limb

5

Dislocation of the sternoclavicular joint

Sprains of the sternoclavicular joint are common, anterior dislocations unusual and posterior dislocations rare. Anterior dislocations have a distinct tendency to become recurrent, 18% in the Mayo Clinic series (Nettles and Linscheid, 1968). Recurrent dislocation causes little disability in most patients, and is only a nuisance to heavy manual workers or weight lifters (Lunseth, Chapman and Frankel, 1975).

Posterior displacement of the inner end of the clavicle may injure vital structures at the root of the neck (Buckerfield and Castle, 1984). Fatal injury has been reported, from rupture of the trachea (Kennedy, 1949). In the absence of such complications the diagnosis of the acute dislocation can be missed (Paterson, 1961), but once reduced the lesion is stable, and heals with thickening of the joint as a residual cosmetic blemish (McKenzie, 1963).

References

Buckerfield, C. T. and Castle, M. E. (1984) Acute traumatic retrosternal dislocation of the clavicle. *Journal of Bone and Joint Surgery,* **66A**, 379–385

Kennedy, J. C. (1949) Retrosternal dislocation of the clavicle. *Journal of Bone and Joint Surgery,* **31B**, 74–75

Lunseth, P. A., Chapman, K. W. and Frankel, V. H. (1975) Surgical treatment of chronic dislocation of the sterno-clavicular joint. *Journal of Bone and Joint Surgery,* **57B**, 193–196

McKenzie, J. M. M. (1963) Retrosternal dislocation of the clavicle. *Journal of Bone and Joint Surgery,* **45B**, 216–218

Nettles, J. L. and Linscheild, R. I. (1968) Sterno-clavicular dislocations. *Journal of Trauma,* **8**, 158–164

Paterson, D. C. (1961) Retrosternal dislocation of the clavicle. *Journal of Bone and Joint Surgery,* **43B**, 90–94

Table 5.1

Injury	Dislocations of the sternoclavicular joint
Structural impairment	*Anterior* – instability leading to recurrence 18% *Posterior* – pressure effects on trachea, great vessels and brachial plexus
Subjective impairment	Pain on heavy lifting
Disability and handicap	Little disability in most patients Heavy manual workers and athletes may be handicapped
Comments	

6
Fractures of the clavicle

Robert Peel, Prime Minister of England, was thrown from his horse on 29th June, 1850, fracturing his clavicle. He died on 2nd July, from a pneumothorax. This is a rare complication of a broken collar bone, an injury seen every day in accident departments. The overwhelming majority heal quickly, but problems do arise and they can be related to the site of fracture. Fractures of the inner end of the clavicle unite without problems, those of the middle third usually do but may leave an ugly lump; fractures of the outer third have an appreciable incidence of non-union, of the order of 35–40%.

Other complications include damage to the brachial plexus or the subclavian vessels. Such lesions clinically dominate the presentation, and prognosis depends on the results of the nervous or arterial injury. Persistent pain has been reported following involvement of cutaneous nerves in the callus of a middle third fracture.

Non-union of the middle third of the clavicle is rare. Neer (1960) found three cases out of 2235 – less than 0.2%. It is so rare that it needs to be distinguished from the even rarer congenital lesion. Congenital pseudarthrosis is nearly always on the right side, except when there is dextrocardia and is significantly associated with cervical rib (Alldred, 1963; Lloyd-Roberts, Apley and Owen, 1975).

References

Alldred, A. J. (1963) Congenital pseudarthrosis of the clavicle. *Journal of Bone and Joint Surgery,* **45B**, 312–319

Lloyd-Roberts, G. C., Apley, A. G. and Owen, R. (1975) Reflections on the aetiology of congenital pseudarthrosis of the clavicle. *Journal of Bone and Joint Surgery,* **57B**, 24–29

Neer, C. S. (1960) Non-union of the clavicle. *Journal of American Medical Association,* **172**, 1006–1011

Table 6.1

Injury	Fractures of the clavicle
Structural impairment	Inner third – none Middle third – malunion almost universal. Remodelling total in children – non-union < 0.2% Outer third – non-union 30–40%. Acromioclavicular osteoarthrosis < 5%
Subjective impairment	
Disability and handicap	With the exception of fractures lateral to the coracoclavicular ligaments, little or no functional disability is to be expected The ugly lump of a malunited clavicular fracture will handicap those whose living depends on their exposed appearance, and those who are self-conscious about their image
Comments	Rare complications include – brachial plexus lesions – subclavian artery damage – pneumothorax – chylothorax

7

Dislocation of the acromioclavicular joint

The residual problems after acromioclavicular injury depend on whether the coraco-acromial ligaments were ruptured in the injury, that is, on whether the lesion is a subluxation or a dislocation. Subluxation leaves a slight prominence of the outer end of the clavicle, causing no functional disability and minimal cosmetic blemish. Dislocation of the joint leaves an ugly protuberance, but again the functional disability is only significant in heavy manual workers. The results of open reduction and fixation are often adversely compared to those of conservative treatment (Larsen, Bjerg-Nielsen and Christensen, 1986), but it must be remembered that operative treatment is usually reserved for those patients who are expected to place heavy demands on their shoulders (Jeffreys, 1985).

Any forecast of the development of post-traumatic osteoarthrosis in the acromioclavicular joint must be made against the knowledge that the joint is frequently affected by degenerative change in young adult life without any history of injury (Worcester and Green, 1968). The reported incidence after injury is 28% (Jacobs and Wade, 1966).

Calcification of the coracoclavicular ligaments is common but does not affect the functional result (Larsen, Bjerg-Nielsen and Christensen, 1986).

A few cases of dislocation of both acromioclavicular and sternoclavicular joints have been reported. The medial dislocation is anterior, the lateral, posterior. The recommended management is to ignore the sternoclavicular lesion and treat the acromioclavicular injury. The results are similar to those reported for isolated acromioclavicular dislocation (Sanders, Lyons and Rockwood, 1990).

References

Jacobs, B. and Wade, P. A. (1966) Acromio-clavicular joint injury. *Journal of Bone and Joint Surgery,* **48A**, 475–486

Jeffreys, T. E. (1985) Carbon Fibre Repair of Acromio-clavicular Dislocation. Instructional Lecture at Oswestry

Larsen, E., Bjerg-Nielsen, A. and Christensen, P. (1986) Conservative or surgical treatment of acromio-clavicular dislocation. *Journal of Bone and Joint Surgery,* **68A**, 552–555

Sanders, J. O., Lyons, F. A. and Rockwood, C. A. (1990) Management of dislocation of both ends of clavicle. *Journal of Bone and Joint Surgery,* **72A**, 399–402

Worcester, J. N. and Green, D. P. (1968) Osteoarthritis of the acromio-clavicular joint. *Clinical Orthopaedics,* **58**, 69–73

Table 7.1

Injury	Dislocation of the acromioclavicular joint
Structural impairment	*Subluxation* – Slight prominence of outer clavicle *Dislocation* – Obvious prominence of outer clavicle – Calcification of coracoclavicular ligaments 40–50% } Osteoarthrosis in 30%
Subjective impairment	Pain and weakness of shoulder in 7–8%
Disability and handicap	Handicap in heavy manual workers Incidence of osteoarthrosis not related to functional result
Comments	Osteolysis of the outer end of the clavicle has been described as a complication, but its relation to the injury is not clear

8

Acute tears of the rotator cuff

Acute full thickness tears of the rotator cuff result in persistent pain and weakness of the shoulder. In a 5-year follow up of such injuries, treated conservatively, it was found that 80% of patients still complained of significant pain. The strength of the shoulder was markedly reduced and half the patients had given up work. Of those still at work only 5% had returned to their pre-accident job. In this series all the patients were manual workers in late middle age (Wallace and Wiley, 1986). Whether operative repair in such patients would have produced significantly better results is doubtful. The reported series of operative repair are largely concerned with younger patients. Moderate relief of pain and moderate restoration of shoulder movement are reported (Bassett and Cofield, 1983).

References

Bassett, R. W. and Cofield, R. H. (1983) Acute tears of the rotator cuff. *Clinical Orthopaedics,* **175**, 18–24

Wallace, W. A. and Wiley, A. M. (1986) Long term results of conservative management of full thickness tears of the rotator cuff. *Journal of Bone and Joint Surgery,* **68B**, 162

Table 8.1

Injury	Acute tears of the rotator cuff
Structural impairment	Full thickness rupture of rotator cuff
Subjective impairment	Pain Weakness Limited movement of shoulder } 80% symptoms at 5 years 76% aware of no change since 6 months after injury 60% reduction of shoulder strength compared to uninjured side
Disability and handicap	54% still at work after 5 years 5% returned to pre-accident employment (Patients under review were manual workers, many near retirement age at the time of injury)
Comments	The reported results of operative repair in young athletes are better

9

Anterior dislocation of the shoulder joint

Traumatic anterior dislocation of the glenohumeral joint can occur at any age, from the moment of delivery onwards. It is an injury which has been extensively discussed, described, and treated by a variety of methods and argued over for centuries. Every individual orthopaedic surgeon has his own views on management. The published results vary wildly in their assessment of the incidence of complications. The most common complication, if not the most serious, is recurrence of dislocation, but there is still disagreement on how to prevent it, if it can be prevented. Descriptions of 'new' operations for the correction of recurrent dislocation appear with monotonous regularity and they all turn out to be variations of an old theme. Small wonder that prognosis in the individual case is inexact and consists of generalizations.

In the elderly a stiff shoulder is more likely to be the residual disability than is instability. Painful ankylosis of a shoulder joint in the elderly can make the difference between dependent and independent daily living.

Other complications include damage to the circumflex nerve, which is common, and to the axillary artery, which is rare. The possible complications may coexist, but, in discussing prognosis, they are best dealt with separately. A combination, as one would expect, affects the outcome adversely.

Recurrence of dislocation ['A lesion peculiar to athletes and epileptics.) (Speed, 1927)]

The overall incidence of recurrence, as reported in the literature, is about 30%, although it is difficult to see how this can be regarded as anything like an accurate estimate. The risk of recurrence decreases with age, almost vanishing in the elderly because the almost inevitable stiffness confers stability. Most

(70%) recurrences happen within 2 years of the initial dislocation, the remainder within 5 years. Recurrence after that time follows a second clear cut injury and is a fresh, initial dislocation.

The factors favouring, or guarding against, recurrence are debatable. 'None of several hundred primary dislocations that I had treated with strict immobilization of the shoulder for at least three weeks had recurred' (Watson-Jones, 1955). There is really no polite answer to that statement. It is generally accepted now that the duration of immobilization is less important than the energy of rehabilitation. It has been said that the more violent injuries are responsible for fewer recurrences. The effect of associated fractures is doubtful. Sex is irrelevant.

Stiffness of the shoulder

The majority of young adults regain normal shoulder function within 4 months. Less than 5% show some residual stiffness. With advancing age the picture changes. Over the age of 40, up to 75% of patients have a varying degree of painful restriction of movement. Improvement can be expected to continue for a year after injury but not longer although no improvement at all by 3 months is ominous. Any delay in reduction dramatically worsens the end result, and this becomes very obvious in the elderly demented whose dislocation may go unrecognized for days or weeks. Much of the residual stiffness in the elderly is due to an associated rotator cuff tear which has been reported as occurring in up to 90% of patients over the age of 40.

Prolonged immobilization in the elderly is counterproductive, as the risk of recurrence is far smaller than the risk of a stiff shoulder. It is interesting to compare the following quotation with Watson-Jones' comment. 'I believe that at present there is too great a tendency to confine the arm after reduction. I believe that uncomplicated cases tend to recover in about four weeks, unless interfered with by injudicious treatment, such as prolonged fixation' (Codman, 1934).

Circumflex nerve injury is seen in up to 30% of all dislocations, with greater frequency in the elderly. Recovery of deltoid function is to be expected, but does not occur in many elderly patients (up to 60%) particularly if there has been delay in reduction. Deltoid contraction should begin within 3 months.

Axillary artery injury is a sufficiently rare complication to be recorded individually. The prognosis depends on prompt diagnosis and access to skilled vascular surgery.

Osteoarthrosis of the shoulder is not seen after promptly reduced primary dislocations. It is a complication of recurrent dislocation and has been reported as occurring in 7% of these patients.

Table 9.1 Results of operations for recurrent anterior dislocation

Surgeon	*Percentage success rate (no further recurrence)*	*Reference*
Bankart	96.7	Rockwood (1984)
Putti–Platt	97	Rockwood (1984)
Magnusson–Stack	95.9	Rockwood (1984)
Bristow	98.3	Rockwood (1984)
Eden–Hybbinette	94	Rockwood (1984)
Du Toit Stapling	97.1	Boyd (1974)

These figures relate to recurrence only and do not take into account residual stiffness. The Putti–Platt operation for example *depends* on restricted external rotation for its success.

References

Boyd, H. B. (1974) In *Campbells Operative Orthopaedics (ed. A. H. Crenshaw), C. V. Mosby, St. Louis, pp. 315–318*

Codman, E. A. (1934) *The Shoulder*, Thomas Todd Company, Boston, p. 283

Rockwood, C. A. (1984) Dislocations of the shoulder. In *Fractures in Adults* (ed. C. A. Rockwood), J. B. Lippincott, Philadelphia

Speed, K. (1927) Recurrent anterior dislocation at the shoulder. *Surgery, Gynaceology and Obstetrics,* **44**, 468–477

Watson-Jones, R. (1955) Fractures and Joint Injuries, 4th edn, Vol. II, E. & S. Livingstone, Edinburgh and London, p. 477

Table 9.2

Injury	Anterior dislocation of the shoulder
Structural impairment	Recurrence – 45–90% (under 20 years) 4–15% (over 40 years) Pain, Stiffness – 60–70% over 40 years Circumflex nerve palsy – 30% Axillary artery lesion – < 1% Osteoarthrosis – 7%
Subjective impairment	Recurrent dislocation Shoulder stiffness – inability to touch back of neck or small of back – inability to elevate above right angle
Disability and handicap	Recurrent dislocation in the young manual worker is incapacitating for work Athletic ability diminished – contact sports precluded Painful stiffness in the elderly may result in total dependency
Comments	Prognosis for recurrence is expectant – 70% recur within 2 years, remainder within 5 years Stiffness present 4–6 months after injury, in the elderly, will be permanent

10

Posterior dislocation of the shoulder

This injury has a reputation for being missed at first presentation. If it is recognized and promptly reduced the results are good, in the young patient. The elderly do badly with persistent pain and stiffness after reduction (Roberts and Wickstrom, 1971). There is a high incidence of recurrence in posterior dislocations, reported from 37 to 60% (Rowe, 1956; Roberts and Wickstrom, 1971).

Late diagnosis can result in surprisingly little disability. The pain of the dislocation settles within a few weeks and the patient is left with a stiff shoulder (Kessel, 1982). Attempting to reduce a dislocation by closed manipulation, which has been present for some weeks, can be dangerous (Codman, 1934). Open reduction has been reported as being successful in maintaining reduction (Hawkins *et al.*, 1987), but other reviews show that the majority of patients so treated have residual pain and limited movement (Rowe and Zarins, 1982). The incidence of osteoarthrosis in late reduction posterior dislocation is thought to be as high as 54%, with the development related to delay in prompt reduction (Samilson and Prieto, 1983).

References

Codman, E. A. (1934) *The Shoulder*, Thomas Todd Company, Boston, p. 292

Hawkins, R. J., Neer, C. S., Pianta, R. M. and Mendoza, F. X. (1987) Locked posterior dislocation of the shoulder. *Journal of Bone and Joint Surgery,* **69A**, 9–18

Kessel, L. (1982) *Clinical Disorders of the Shoulder*, Churchill Livingstone, Edinburgh and London

Roberts, A. and Wickstrom, J. (1971) Prognosis of posterior dislocation of shoulder. *Acta Orthopaedica Scandinavia,* **42**, 328–337

Rowe, C. R. (1956) Prognosis in dislocations of the shoulder. *Journal of Bone and Joint Surgery,* **38A**, 957–977

Rowe, C. R. and Zarins, B. (1982) Chronic unreduced dislocations of the shoulder. *Journal of Bone and Joint Surgery,* **64A**, 494–505

Samilson, R. L. and Prieto, V. (1983) Dislocation arthropathy of the shoulder. *Journal of Bone and Joint Surgery,* **64A**, 456–460

Table 10.1

Injury	Posterior dislocations of the shoulder
Structural impairment	*Immediate reduction* – no residual impairment in the young 37–60% recurrence *Chronic dislocation* – Osteoarthrosis? 54% (no accurate assessment published)
Subjective impairment	Chronic dislocation. Pain (of short duration) Stiffness
Disability and handicap	Chronic dislocation produces little disability in the elderly
Comments	The incidence of post-traumatic osteoarthrosis is related to the delay in diagnosis and reduction. After late open reduction over 50% have residual pain and restricted elevation of the shoulder

11

Fractures of the neck of the humerus

In 1934, E. A. Codman wrote about fractures of the upper end of the humerus 'most cases eventually recover pretty good use of their shoulders in spite of any kind of treatment. Only those in which the displacement is very great or in which the treatment is neglected very grossly (perhaps by the patient) result in ankylosis' (Codman, 1934). He also observed that displaced 'two part' fractures had a worse prognosis than undisplaced 'four part' fractures. His principles of classification as a guide to prognosis remained largely ignored until Neer's (1970) re-emphasis of classification. Codman's classic book is imperative reading for those interested in injuries of the shoulder.

More recent reviews have confirmed Codman's emphasis on displacement being the key to prognosis. Neer (1970) distinguished between displaced and undisplaced fractures in his 'two, three and four part fractures'. Stableforth (1984) found severe pain, stiffness and functional disability common after conservatively managed four part fractures. Only one of his cases was free of pain and half them were dependent on assistance in daily living. Clifford (1980) found undisplaced fractures to do well with over 90% having excellent or good function 18 months after injury. He identified displacement of the fragments as being responsible for a poor result, but also identified prolonged immobilization and prolonged physiotherapy as associated factors. The incrimination of physiotherapy is perhaps a little unjust as severely injured shoulders inevitably need more physiotherapy (Clifford, 1980). Stableforth (1984) stressed the importance of skilled physiotherapy in obtaining optimal function. His conclusion, based on a retrospective comparative review, was that the prognosis for displaced four part fractures was so poor that they should be managed by primary prosthetic replacement.

References

Clifford, P. C. (1980) Fractures of the neck of the humerus: a review of the late results. *Injury,* **12**, 21–25

Codman, E. A. (1934) *The Shoulder*, Thomas Todd Company, Boston, p. 331

Neer, C. S. (1970) Displaced proximal humeral fractures. *Journal of Bone and Joint Surgery,* **52A**, 1077–1089

Stableforth, P. G. (1984) Four part fractures of the neck of the humerus. *Journal of Bone and Joint Surgery,* **66B**, 104–108

Table 11.1

Injury	Fractures of the neck of the humerus: undisplaced
Structural impairment	Malunion – absent or minimal by definition Non-union – not recorded Avascular necrosis – 'high' in fractures of anatomical neck (Neer) Glenohumeral osteoarthrosis – uncommon, ankylosis more often result of extra-articular adhesion
Subjective impairment	Pain Stiffness – inability to reach mouth or buttock } Less than 10%
Disability and handicap	The disability of a stiff and painful shoulder is increased if the dominant limb is affected. Handicap in daily living includes activities such as personal toilet, eating, driving Occupational handicap affects skilled craftsmen and mechanics as well as manual workers
Comments	Although overall end results are good (over 90%) full recovery may be prolonged to 18 months. Overlong immobilization delays recovery

Table 11.2

Injury	Fractures of the proximal humerus: displaced (two, three and four part)
Structural impairment	Malunion – almost 100% with conservative management Non-union – 23% (Neer) particularly in avulsion of greater tuberosity Avascular necrosis – 6–25% (average 10%) (75% in 4 part fractures) Brachial plexus lesion – 6% in 4 part fractures
Subjective impairment	Pain Stiffness
Disability and handicap	2 Part: 20% poor result. 3 Part: 40% poor result. 4 Part: 50% loss of independence Nearly 100% with significant disability. A significant number (up to 50%) became dependent for daily living. Overall results for return to heavy manual work poor. Skilled workers also significantly handicapped
Comments	The prognosis becomes worse as the extent of comminution, and degree of displacement, of the fragment increase Primary prosthetic replacement advocated for 4 part fractures

Fracture separations of proximal humeral epiphysis

I have never seen an adult with residual disability from this injury, in over 30 years of orthopaedic practice.

12 Fractures of the shaft of the humerus

Most fractures of the humeral shaft are uncomplicated and unite readily with acceptable degrees of malunion. 'Few injuries are more easy to treat. Union of most of these fractures is so rapid that it is difficult to stop' (Watson-Jones, 1955). A return to normal function within 6–9 months can be predicted for 90% of patients. A few do badly. Delayed or non-union occurs in up to 10% of cases; the reviews give various incidences ranging from 1% (Thompson *et al.*, 1965) to 15% (Mast *et al.*, 1975). The definition of delayed union is also variable. Watson-Jones (1955) wrote that mobility 'almost as free as at the time of injury' at the fourth or fifth week was ominous, while Klenerman (1966) regarded the presence of movement at 8 weeks as being evidence of delayed union. There are few indicators to the likelihood of delayed union. The incidence of delayed and non-union decreases with the level of the fracture (Klenerman, 1966). Transverse fractures are more likely to be delayed in union than comminuted or long oblique fractures. Compound fractures will be associated with delay if the wound is extensive and if there has been stripping of soft tissue from the fragments.

Radial nerve palsy, associated with closed fractures, can be neurapraxia. Neurapraxia is an incomplete lesion and recovery is certain. Thorough neurological examination will show evidence of 'escape', and when this is found, spontaneous recovery of radial nerve function can be predicted confidently. When radial nerve lesions are associated with compound fractures it is possible that the structural continuity of the nerve has been interrupted. Exploration of the nerve is then indicated. In closed fractures an adequate time can be as long as 9 months (Seddon, 1942; Pollock *et al.*, 1981).

A new type of nerve lesion has been described when demyelinization follows pressure on a peripheral nerve trunk. The lesion has been termed 'axonamonosis'. One reported case occurred in association with a closed fracture of the shaft of the humerus. Operative decompression was followed by rapid and complete recovery (Birch and Strange, 1990).

Malunion after conservatively treated humeral shaft fractures is common; it is not usually gross and has little or no effect on final function. Shortening is not significant in the arm, and up to 30° of varus bowing is compatible with normal function (Klenerman, 1966; Hunter, 1982).

References

Birch, R. and Strange, F. G. St. C. (1990) A new type of peripheral nerve lesion. *Journal of Bone and Joint Surgery,* **72B**, 312–313

Hunter, S. G. (1982) The closed treatment of humeral fractures. *Clinical Orthopaedics,* **164**, 192–198

Klenerman, L. (1966) Fractures of the shaft of the humerus. *Journal of Bone and Joint Surgery,* **48B**, 105–111

Mast, J. W., Spiegel, P. G., Harvey, J. P. and Harrison, C. (1975) Fractures of the humeral shaft. *Clinical Orthopaedics,* **112**, 254–262

Pollock, F. H., Drake, D., Bovill, E. G., Day, L. and Trafton, P. G. (1981) Treatment of radial neuropathy associated with fractures of the humerus. *Journal of Bone and Joint Surgery,* **63A**, 239–243

Seddon, H. J. (1942) A classification of nerve injuries. *British Medical Journal,* **II**, 237–239

Thompson, R. G., Compere, E. L., Schnute, W. J., Compere, C. L., Kernahan, W. T. and Keagy, R. D. (1965) The treatment of humeral shaft fractures by the hanging cast method. *Journal of International College of Surgeons,* **43**, 52–60

Watson-Jones, R. (1955) *Fractures and Joint Injuries*, 4th edn, Vol. II, E. & S. Livingstone, Edinburgh and London, p. 503

Table 12.1

Injury	Fractures of shaft of humerus
Structural impairment	Malunion. Shortening. Varus angulation. Anterior angulation Non-union. Proximal one-third 11–17%. Middle one-third 8–11%. Lower one-third 5–6% Radial nerve palsy. Proximal one-third 5%. Middle one-third 12–15%. Lower one third 20–30%
Subjective impairment	Normal function in up to 90% of uncomplicated fractures
Disability and handicap	Varus or anterior angulation less than 30%, lateral displacement, or shortening of 2 cm do not result in disability. 80–90% achieve normal function. Results of treatment of non-union variable. Best results achieved by compression plating and grafting
Comments	Radial nerve lesion in closed fractures is in continuity. Recovery may not begin for 9 months. Exploration should be delayed until then

13

Fractures of the lower end of the humerus in adults

Supracondylar fractures of the humerus do not involve the articular surface of the elbow joint, and, if they unite, the functional result is satisfactory, even with some degree of malunion (Aitken and Rorabeck, 1986; Browne, O'Riordan and Quinlan, 1986). There is a low incidence of non-union, which, even if successfully treated, is associated with a stiff elbow and residual disability in 65% of cases (Ackerman and Jupiter, 1988).

Intercondylar fractures, often comminuted, and intra-articular fractures, have a bad reputation, with over 90% of patients being left with a stiff and painful elbow (Watson-Jones, 1955; Zagorski *et al.*, 1986). Open reduction and fixation on Association Osteosynthesis (Swiss) (AO) principles can transform this gloomy prognosis, with good results in 80% of treated cases being reported (Shetty, 1982).

The incidence of post-traumatic osteoarthrosis is 62% and this high incidence is not affected by the accuracy of the reduction (Jupiter *et al.*, 1985). The arthrotic changes were mild in 52.9%, and severe in 8.8%. The severity of the radiological changes did not correlate with the functional results which were excellent in nearly 80% of these 34 cases. The three cases with marked degenerative changes experienced no pain and slight limitation of movement, at 2.5–3 years after injury. The arthrosis may progress with time, with diminished movement and pain becoming apparent over 10 years later.

References

Ackerman, G. and Jupiter, J. B. (1988) Non-union of fracture of the distal end of the humerus. *Journal of Bone and Joint Surgery,* **70A**, 75–83

Aitken, G. K. and Rorabeck, C. H. (1986) Distal humeral fractures in the adult. *Clinical Orthopaedics,* **207**, 191–197

Browne, A. O., O'Riordan, M. and Quinlan, W. (1986) Supracondylar fractures of the humerus in adults. *Injury,* **17**, 184–186

Jupiter, J. B., Neff, U., Holzack, P. and Allgower, M. (1985) Intercondylar fracture of the humerus. *Journal of Bone and Joint Surgery,* **67A**, 226–239

Shetty, S. (1982) Surgical treatment of T and Y fractures of the distal humerus. *Injury,* **14**, 345–348

Watson-Jones, R. (1955) *Fractures and Joint Injuries*, 4th edn, Vol II, E. & S. Livingstone, Edinburgh and London, pp. 534–536

Zagorski, J. B., Jennings, J. J., Burkhalter, W. E. and Uribe, J. W. (1986) Comminuted intra-articular fractures of the distal humeral condyles. *Clinical Orthopaedics,* **202**, 197–204

Table 13.1

Injury	Supracondylar fractures of the humerus in adults
Structural impairment	Malunion Non-union 2%
Subjective impairment	Symptoms associated with non-union are stiffness, instability and pain
Disability and handicap	Disability from non-union can be profound, even after successful treatment of non-union
Comments	

Table 13.2

Injury	Intercondylar fractures of the humerus in adults
Structural impairment	Malunion – over 80% Osteoarthrosis – 68%
Subjective impairment	Pain, Stiffness } In 20.5%
Disability and handicap	Restricted extension of the elbow in itself inflicts little handicap, even in manual workers. Painful restriction, however, results in significant disability
Comments	Prognosis can be reversed by anatomical reduction and internal fixation. The incidence of osteoarthrosis is little changed but a good functional result is to be expected in 80%

14

Supracondylar fractures of the humerus in children

This fracture has, rightly, acquired the reputation of being more responsible for Volkmann's ischaemic contracture than any other. In the western world that complication nowadays is rare (0.5%), but its avoidance has perhaps led to a greater acceptance of residual varus deformity of the elbow. The overall results are excellent or good in over 90% of children (Henrickson, 1966). The best results follow perfect reduction of the fracture (Watson-Jones, 1955; Warlock and Colton, 1987). When union has occurred the potential for persistent varus deformity can be measured by Baumann's angle, sub-tended by lines drawn along the vertical axis of the humerus and the plane of the lateral condylar growth plate. This angle is to be compared with the corresponding angle in the uninjured elbow. Residual varus is associated with loss or reversal of the carrying angle. Neurapraxia of the median and radial nerves has a reported incidence of 10% (Thomas and Alpar, 1987).

References

Henrickson, B. (1966) Supra-condylar fractures of the elbow in children. *Acta Chirurgica Scandinavia* (Supplement), 369

Thomas, A. P. and Alpar, E. K. (1987) Outcome of supra-condylar fractures of the humerus in children. *Journal of the Royal Society of Medicine*, **80**, 347–351

Warlock, P. H. and Colton, C. L. (1987) Severely displaced supra-condylar fractures of the humerus in children. *Journal of Paediatric Orthopaedics*, **7**, 49–53

Watson-Jones, R. (1955) *Fractures and Joint Injuries*, 4th edn, Vol. II, E. & S. Livingstone, Edinburgh, p. 525

Table 14.1

Injury	Supracondylar fractures of the humerus in children
Structural impairment	Malunion. Residual cubitus varus. Deformity may increase with growth Ischaemic contracture of flexor muscles. Less than 0.5% Nerve lesions – 7%. Radial most often affected. Complete recovery expected Osteoarthrosis of elbow joint – 2%
Subjective impairment	*Cubitus varus*. Unsightly but functional disability only if varus more than 25° *Limited flexion* due to imperfect reduction of posteriorly displaced lower fragment *Ischaemic contracture* produces clawing of fingers and median nerve anaesthesia. The functional disability is crippling
Disability and handicap	Varies from nil to severe with degree of deformity
Comments	The best results follow perfect reduction with no vascular or nervous impairment The extent of initial displacement only influences prognosis if perfect reduction is not achieved; in itself it does not affect prognosis

15

Fractures of the lateral humeral condyle in children

Few injuries in childhood have greater potential for complication than this. The fractured segment includes three ossific centres. Return to normal function within 3 months is to be expected (Badger, 1954; Wilkins, 1984), but late complications abound, of which tardy ulnar palsy is the best known. The onset of ulnar nerve problems may be delayed until adult life, but can occur within 8 years (Jakob *et al.*, 1975). Wadsworth (1964, 1972) has detailed the possible complications. They include non-union, malunion (overgrowth), premature epiphyseal fusion, avascular necrosis and ulnar neuritis, which is usually but not always the sequel of cubitus valgus. The problems are said to be prevented by prompt open reduction and fixation. In cases seen later the results of open reduction have been found to be no better than in untreated cases (Jakob *et al.*, 1975). The undisplaced cases in this series all did well, but Jeffery (1958) found that 10 out of 13 cases of non-union occurred in undisplaced fractures treated conservatively. Wadsworth (1964) found two cases of premature fusion in eight undisplaced fractures. Prognosis must be guarded even in the undisplaced fractures and Jeffery advised repeated radiographic review over a period of a year after injury, to exclude non-union.

The residual valgus of non-union or premature fusion does not result in any disability, but the deformity is ugly and this may well be a handicap in certain occupations, to the point of disqualifying a recruit to the armed forces for example. Delayed ulnar palsy can cause distressing symptoms as well as the more disabling motor weakness of a high ulnar nerve lesion. There is an unknown incidence of osteoarthrosis of the elbow following this fracture.

References

Badger, F. G. (1954) Fractures of the lateral humeral condyle. *Journal of Bone and Joint Surgery,* **36B**, 147–148

Jakob, R., Fowles, J. V., Rang, M. and Kassab, M. T. (1975) Observations concerning fractures of the lateral humeral condyle in children. *Journal of Bone and Joint Surgery,* **57B**, 430–436

Jeffery, C. C. (1958) Non-union of the epiphysis of the lateral condyle of the humerus. *Journal of Bone and Joint Surgery,* **40B**, 397–405

Wadsworth, T. G. (1964) Premature epiphyseal fusion after injury of the capitellum. *Journal of Bone and Joint Surgery,* **46B**, 46–49

Wadsworth, T. G. (1972) Injuries of the lateral humeral condylar epiphysis. *Clinical Orthopaedics,* **85**, 127–142

Wilkins, K. E. (1984) Fractures and dislocations in the elbow region. In *Fractures in Children*, Vol. 3 (eds C. A. Rockwood, K. E. Wilkins and R. E. King), J. B. Lippincott, Philadelphia

Table 15.1

Injury	Fractures of the lateral condyle in children
Structural impairment	*Early* Malunion 25% Non-union 16% Avascular necrosis 23% Premature fusion 20% *Late* Cubitus valgus Ulnar neuropathy Osteoarthrosis of elbow
Subjective impairment	The symptoms of ulnar neuropathy can be delayed in onset until adult life but have been reported within 8 years of injury
Disability and handicap	Valgus deformity alone does not consititute a disability, but may be such a cosmetic blemish as to disqualify for certain occupations
Comments	Prompt open reduction has been advocated to prevent late complications, but they occur with undisplaced fractures and after skilfully treated displaced fractures. Open reduction of late cases does not produce any better results than untreated cases, but anterior transposition of the ulnar nerve is advised

16

Displacement of the epiphysis of the medial epicondyle

This is an avulsion injury of the common flexor origin and the epicondylar fragment is displaced, the degree of displacement being an index of the degree of valgus force. Increasing displacement is associated with ulnar nerve damage. Recovery from this lesion is good but delayed ulnar neuritis can follow non-union of the fragment. A long-term review found a 55% incidence of non-union with 10% of these patients experiencing ulnar nerve symptoms (Josefsson and Danielsson, 1986).

Reference

Josefsson, P. O. and Danielsson, L. G. (1986) Epicondylar elbow fracture in children. *Acta Orthopaedica Scandinavia,* **57**, 313–315

Table 16.1

Injury	Fractures of the medial epicondyle
Structural impairment	Non-union. 55% of displaced fragments Ulnar nerve lesion in 10% of non-unions
Subjective impairment	
Disability and handicap	Non-union produces little or no disability, the strength and range of elbow movement being unaffected Ulnar nerve lesions present in later life, with impaired hand function
Comments	

17

Injuries around the elbow

Common to most elbow injuries in adults is the sequel of restricted movement, particularly extension. The loss of full extension is hardly a disability, but a restriction of more than 45% is.

Other complications common to most elbow injuries involving the articular surface are:

1. Osteoarthrosis.
2. Myositis ossificans.
3. Loose body formation.
4. Tardy ulnar palsy.

Osteoarthrosis of the elbow

Even when regarded as idiopathic, this occurs most commonly in the dominant arm of manual workers and can fairly be regarded as having an occupational, probably traumatic, origin. The radiographic appearances may be quite striking and out of proportion to the symptoms and signs. The patient is usually unaware of the lost extension that is revealed by examination. Pain is caused either by a loose body, or persists after a minor strain. Presentation can be acute with 'locking' of the joint or with a haemarthrosis.

Myositis ossificans

This is the formation of new bone in soft tissue. It can occur in the absence of trauma (Hardy and Dickson, 1963; Jeffreys and Stiles, 1966), but usually presents as a complication of major bony injury particularly around the elbow joint. It is more common in children than in adults. Predisposing factors have been identified as the severity of injury producing soft tissue and periosteal stripping, over-zealous manipulation, and forced passive movement of a stiff joint (Thompson and Garcia, 1967). The heterotropic bone matures with time, becoming discrete and encapsulated.

Loose bodies

Loose bodies in the elbow joint can arise in two ways. Bony fragments, particularly after fractures of the radial head, may end up in the joint cavity. When a radial head is excised, the fragments must be assembled to ensure that no fragments are missing. Loose bodies of cartilage and bone can be shed by the synovium of an osteoarthrotic joint.

Ulnar palsy

This classically follows the cubitus valgus that follows lateral condylar fractures in childhood, but can also be produced by osteophytic outgrowth of the humero-ulnar margins (Wadsworth, 1972).

References

Hardy, A. G. and Dickson, J. W. (1963) Pathological ossification in traumatic paraplegia. *Journal of Bone and Joint Surgery,* **45B**, 76–79

Jeffreys, T. E. and Stiles, P. J. (1966) Pseudomalignant osseous tumour of soft tissue. *Journal of Bone and Joint Surgery,* **48B**, 488–492

Thompson, H. C. and Garcia, A. (1967) Myositis ossificans. Aftermath of elbow injuries. *Clinical Orthopaedics,* **50**, 129–134

Wadsworth, T. G. (1972) Injuries of the capitular epiphysis. *Clinical Orthopaedics,* **85**, 127–142

18

Fractures of the olecranon

These are intra-articular fractures and their prognosis regarding joint movement, and the later development of osteoarthrosis of the elbow joint, depends on the quality of their reduction (Helm, Hornby and Miller, 1987; Holdsworth and Mossad, 1984; Kiviluoto and Santavirta, 1978). They are also disruptions of the extensor apparatus at the elbow, the olecranon being the analogue of the patella, and some weakness of elbow extension may result (Holdsdworth and Mossad, 1984). Secure fixation allows rehabilitation to be prompt; union is rapid and in the majority of patients normal function is regained within 3 months (Helm, Hornby and Miller, 1987; Wadsworth, 1976). If the initial injury is particularly severe and the olecranon fracture is complicated by other injuries around the elbow, the incidence of late osteoarthrosis rises to nearly 80% (Morris *et al.*, 1978).

References

Helm, R. H., Hornby, R. and Miller, S. W. M. (1987) The complications of surgical treatment of displaced fractures of the olecranon. *Injury,* **18,** 48–50

Holdsworth, B. J. and Mossad, M. M. (1984) Elbow function following tension band fixation of displaced olecranon fractures. *Injury,* **16**, 182–187

Kiviluoto, O. and Santavirta, S. (1978) Fractures of the olecranon. *Acta Orthopaedica Scandinavia,* **49**, 28–31

Morris, E. W., Miller, J. H., McLatchie, G. R. and Amis, A. (1978) Combined forces injury of the elbow joint. *Journal of Bone and Joint Surgery,* **60B**, 444

Wadsworth, T. G. (1976) Screw fixation of the olecranon. *Lancet,* **ii**, 118

Table 18.1

Injury	Fractures of the olecranon
Structural impairment	Malunion, after displaced fractures. Dependent on accuracy of reduction/fixation Non-union 3% Osteoarthrosis 2–20% dependent on 1. severity of injury, 2. accuracy of reduction
Subjective impairment	Painful stiffness of elbow joint Limited ability to reach head and neck, back and buttocks
Disability and handicap	Activities of daily living, including personal toilet, affected by limited movement Skilled craftsmen affected more than manual workers
Comments	Good results are claimed for different methods of internal fixation but some loss of extension (up to 30°) reported with all

19

Fractures of the head of the radius

Undisplaced fractures of the head of the radius do well with simple splintage and aspiration of the haemarthrosis (Pinder, 1969; Fleetcroft, 1984). There is controversy regarding the management of displaced fractures. Left undisturbed, an acceptable range of movement results (Jeffreys and Hooker, 1962, unpublished data; Miller, Brennan and Maylahn, 1981; Mathur and Sharma, 1984). Osteoarthrotic change with progressive pain and stiffness are common late sequelae (Goldberg, Peylon and Yosipovitch, 1986; Holdsworth, Clement and Rothwell, 1987). The results of excision, however, are not satisfactory, with subluxation of the inferior radio-ulnar joint causing pain or weakness at the wrist in 30–50% of patients (Taylor and O'Connor, 1964; Mikic and Vukadinovic, 1983). Late cubitus valgus after radial head excision may lead to tardy ulnar palsy (Mikic and Vukadinovic, 1983). This has lead many surgeons to advocate prosthetic replacement, but the reported results vary widely with a 30% failure rate in one review (Morrey, Askew and Chao, 1981).

References

Fleetcroft, J. P. (1984) Fractures of the radial head. *Journal of Bone and Joint Surgery,* **66B**, 141–142

Goldberg, I., Peylon, J. and Yosipovitch, Z. (1986) Late results of excision of the radial head. *Journal of Bone and Joint Surgery,* **68A**, 675–679

Holdsworth, J. B., Clement, D. A. and Rothwell, P. N. R. (1987) Fractures of the radial head. *Injury,* **18**, 44–47

Mathur, N. and Sharma, C. S. (1984) Fractures of the head of the radius treated by elbow cast. *Acta Orthopaedica Scandinavia,* **55**, 567–568

Mikic, Z. D. and Vukadinovic, S. M. (1983) Late results in fractures of the radial head treated by excision. *Clinical Orthopaedics,* **181**, 220–228

Miller, G. K., Brennan, D. B. and Maylahn, D. J. (1981) Treatment of displaced segmental radial head fractures. *Journal of Bone and Joint Surgery,* **63A**, 712–717

Morrey, B. F., Askew, L. and Chao, Y. (1981) Silastic prosthetic replacement for the radial head. *Journal of Bone and Joint Surgery,* **63A**, 63–68
Pinder, I. M. (1969) Fracture of the head of the radius in adults. *Journal of Bone and Joint Surgery,* **51B**, 386
Taylor, T. K. F. and O'Connor, B. T. (1964) The effect on the inferior radio-ulnar joint of excision of the head of the radius in adults. *Journal of Bone and Joint Surgery,* **46B**, 83–88

Table 19.1

Injury	Fractures of the head of the radius
Structural impairment	*Undisplaced fractures* have up to 95% good results *Displaced and comminuted fractures* – malunion by definition – osteoarthrosis 85–100%
Subjective impairment	Painful restriction of elbow and forearm movement No correlation between radiographic change and symptoms Stiffness progressive over years
Disability and handicap	Less than 20° loss of extension inflicts no handicap Greater loss of movement imposes progressively more severe handicap
Comments	Excision of the radial head, immediate or delayed, with or without prosthetic replacement, is the recommended management for displaced fractures. Complications of excision reported as – weakness 7%, stiffness 25–50%; radio-ulnar subluxation 40–65%, but symptomatic in 30% Ulnar neuritis – following cubitus valgus 5–8%

20
Dislocation of the elbow (in adults)

Most elbow dislocations are posterior fracture dislocations. Residual loss of extension is inevitable, its amount being related to the duration of immobilization after reduction (Protzman, 1978). Peri-articular calcification is common but does not affect elbow movement (Joseffson, Johnell and Gentz, 1984). Post-traumatic osteoarthrosis is seen in over one-third of patients (Joseffson, Johnell and Gentz, 1984). Recurrent dislocation has been reported (Osborne and Cotterill, 1966).

References

Joseffson, P. O., Johnell, O. and Gentz, C. F. (1984) Long term sequelae of simple dislocation of the elbow. *Journal of Bone and Joint Surgery,* **66A**, 927–930

Osborne, G. and Cotterill, P. (1966) Recurrent dislocation of the elbow. *Journal of Bone and Joint Surgery,* **48B**, 340–346

Protzman, R. R. (1978) Dislocation of the elbow joint. *Journal of Bone and Joint Surgery,* **60A**, 539–541

Table 20.1

Injury	Dislocation of the elbow in adults
Structural impairment	Periarticular calcification – 60% Osteoarthrosis of the elbow – 38–40% (may be delayed in onset up to 20 years)
Subjective impairment	Some loss of extension inevitable (average 12–15%) Residual pain has been reported as present in 45% at 34 months
Disability and handicap	Manual workers are not usually handicapped by a stiff elbow until the stiffness is accompanied by pain. Loss of extension of up to 20° imposes no disability
Comments	Osteoarthrosis of the elbow is a common late sequel of elbow injuries. It may cause little disability and present only when loose bodies lock the joint, or after further minor injury

21

Fractures of the upper radial epiphysis

In young children quite considerable degrees of displacement will remodel fully, leaving no clinical or radiological abnormality after healing has occurred. Jeffery (1950) found that up to 60% of tilt would be so corrected in children under 5 years of age. He advised that an angulation greater than this should be corrected at any age. The older is the child the less is the potential for remodelling. Total displacement, with the radial head rotated 90° to be parallel with the radial shaft, will inevitably result in premature fusion of the epiphysis, with deformity of the head and slight restriction of movement. This occurred in three of Jeffery's 24 patients (12.5%). Growth rate discrepancy may then result in cubitus valgus and tardy ulnar palsy in adult life.

Reference

Jeffery, C. C. (1950) Fractures of the head of the radius in children. *Journal of Bone and Joint Surgery,* **32B**, 314–324

Table 21.1

Injury	Fractures of upper radial epiphysis
Structural impairment	Remodelling should correct deformity of 60° under 5 years, 15° in prepuberty Complete displacement produces premature closure of epiphysis and deformity of head and radius. Cubitus valgus may follow
Subjective impairment	Slight restriction of movement not noticed by child
Disability and handicap	Ulnar nerve lesion in adult life if cubitus valgus pronounced
Comments	

22

Dislocation of the elbow in children

Posterior dislocation of the elbow in children may be associated with separation of the medial humeral epicondyle. When this happens the ulnar nerve can be injured. The incidence of nerve damage has been reported as 11% (Wilkins, 1984). Myositis ossificans and recurrence of dislocation occur infrequently (Thompson and Garcia, 1967). Major vascular lesions are rare.

References

Thompson, H. C. and Garcia, A. (1967) Myositis ossificans. Aftermath of elbow injuries. *Clinical Orthopaedics,* **50**, 129–134

Wilkins, K. E. (1984) *Fractures in Children*, Vol. 3 (eds C. A. Rockwood, K. E. Wilkins and R. E. King), J. B. Lippincott, Philadelphia

Table 22.1

Injury	Dislocation of the elbow in children
Structural impairment	Recurrence – 0.7% Ulnar nerve lesion – 11% Arterial injury – rare Myositis ossificans – 3–18% (higher incidence with fracture dislocation)
Subjective impairment	
Disability and handicap	No residual disability in the uncomplicated case
Comments	

23

Fractures of radius and ulna (in adults)

The radius and ulna and the superior and inferior radio-ulnar joints make up a closed ring system. Successful rotation of the forearm depends on that system being intact; any displacement of one of its components will impose restriction of movement of the ring. Equally, displacement can only occur if two segments of the ring are broken. Isolated displaced fractures of the radius are accompanied, perforce, by dislocation of the inferior radio-ulnar joint, the Galeazzi fracture dislocation. Isolated displaced fractures of the ulna are accompanied by dislocation of the superior radio-ulnar joint, the Monteggia fracture dislocation. Displaced fractures of the lower radius are accompanied by fractures of the styloid process of the ulna, the Colles' or Barton's fractures. The exception to this rule are fractures of the olecranon above the level of the superior radio-ulnar articulation. At this level these fractures are to be regarded as disruptions of the extensor mechanism of the elbow, discrete from the rotational injuries of the forearm.

It follows that restoration of normal forearm movement, that is to say, of full pronation and supination, depends on union in anatomical alignment. Anything less must impair movement. The difficulty of obtaining this perfect alignment, although not beyond achievement, has led to these fractures being treated by open reduction and internal fixation whenever the circumstances permit. As always, open operation has its own complications, of delayed and non-union, of infection and of cross union. Functionally satisfactory results can be reached by the enthusiastic application of conservative principles (Sarmiento, Cooper and Sinclair, 1975). In this series the non-union rate is quoted as 2%, malunion as 4.5% and restricted rotation of significant degree in 4.5% of treated cases. Union of both fractures occurred, on average, in 15 weeks. The published results of internal fixation must be judged against this background (Hicks, 1961; Burwell and

Charnley, 1964; Hadden, Reschauer and Segl, 1983). The non-union rate in Hicks' series was 6%, with Burwell and Charnley 2.2%, and using the AO technique 2.8% overall. These are excellent results but carry an infection rate of 2.5%.

References

Burwell, H. N. and Charnley, A. D. (1964) Treatment of forearm fractures in adults with particular reference to plate fixation. *Journal of Bone and Joint Surgery,* **46B**, 404–425

Hadden, W. A., Reschauer, R. and Segl, W. (1983) Results of A.O. plate fixation of forearm shaft fractures in adults. *Injury,* **15**, 44–52

Hicks, J. H. (1961) Fractures of the forearm treated by rigid fixation. *Journal of Bone and Joint Surgery,* **43B**, 680–687

Sarmiento, A., Cooper, J. S. and Sinclair, W. F. (1975) Forearm fractures: early functional bracing. *Journal of Bone and Joint Surgery,* **57A**, 297–304

Table 23.1

Injury	Fractures of both bones of forearm in adults
Structural impairment	Malunion – up to 10%. Synostosis 2% Non-union – up to 10% Delayed union – up to 20%. Prolonged immobilization leads to restricted rotation in 40–60%
Subjective impairment	Restricted rotation of forearm
Disability and handicap	To some extent, loss of pronation and supination can be compensated by shoulder movement, but loss of screwing and turning functions of the hand will interfere with the working ability of skilled craftsmen and mechanics
Comments	The unsatisfactory results of conservative treatment has led to ORIF being the treatment of choice. Operative treatment is reported to have 97% good results (but with a 2.5% infection rate)

24

Fracture of the shaft of the ulna with dislocation of the superior radio-ulnar joint

Monteggia's fracture dislocation fulfils the dictum that one forearm bone cannot be displaced without the ring system giving way at another point. A satisfactory functional result can only occur if both elements of the injury are reduced. This may be achieved by closed methods of treatment (Evans, 1949; Watson-Jones, 1955), but the present consensus is to treat these injuries by open reduction and internal fixation (ORIF), except, possibly, in children (Bruce, Harvey and Wilson, 1974; Reckling, 1982; Wiley and Galey, 1985).

The diagnosis of a Monteggia fracture dislocation is sometimes missed. The problem may be brought to light after further minor trauma, when the original lesion is recognized. It may then be regarded as a congenital dislocation of the radial head. The very existence of such a lesion is questioned by some authorities (Lloyd-Roberts and Bucknill, 1977).

There is an appreciable incidence of nerve injury associated with the Monteggia fracture. The lesion is usually a neurapraxia, with recovery of function within 3 months (Spar, 1977; Wiley and Galey, 1985). Delayed palsy of the posterior interosseous nerve has been reported (Austin, 1976).

Watson-Jones (1955) gives a formidable list of possible complications of the Monteggia fracture dislocation. Apart from unreduced dislocation of the radial head (which should now be of historical import only), he mentions myositis ossificans, cross union between radius and ulna, dislocation of the lower end of the ulna following premature excision of the head of the radius, and non-union of the ulna.

References

Austin, R. (1976) Tardy palsy of the radial nerve from a Monteggia fracture. *Injury*, **7**, 202–204

Bruce, H. E., Harvey, J. P. and Wilson, J. C. (1974) Monteggia fracture. *Journal of Bone and Joint Surgery,* **56A**, 1563–1576

Evans, E. M. (1949) Pronation injuries of the forearm. *Journal of Bone and Joint Surgery,* **31B**, 579–584

Lloyd-Roberts, G. C. and Bucknill, T. M. (1977) Anterior dislocation of the radial head in children. *Journal of Bone and Joint Surgery,* **59B**, 402–407

Reckling, F. W. (1982) Unstable fracture-dislocations of the forearm. *Journal of Bone and Joint Surgery,* **64A**, 857–863

Spar, I. (1977) A neurologic complication following Monteggia fracture. *Clinical Orthopaedics,* **122**, 207–209

Wiley, J. J. and Galey, J. P. (1985) Monteggia injuries in children. *Journal of Bone and Joint Surgery,* **67B**, 728–731

Watson-Jones, R. (1955) Monteggia fracture-dislocation. In *Fractures and Joint Injuries*, 4th edn, Vol. II, E. & S. Livingstone, Edinburgh and London, pp. 572–581

Table 24.1

Injury	Monteggia fracture dislocation
Structural impairment	Unreduced displacement of the head of the radius leaves a deformed elbow, with limited elbow movement and forearm rotation
Subjective impairment	
Disability and handicap	Results of treatment are excellent in over 90% of children, but less than 50% in adults
Comments	Unreduced dislocation of the radial head must be distinguished from congenital dislocation There is a 16% incidence of neurapraxia, usually of radial nerve

25

Fracture of the shaft of the radius with inferior radio-ulnar dislocation

Galeazzi's fracture dislocation is an unstable injury and there is a high incidence of redisplacement after closed reduction. The disability which follows malunion is considerable, both forearm rotation and wrist movement being restricted. Preservation of radial length by open reduction and internal fixation produces a satisfactory functional result (Moore *et al.*, 1985).

Reference

Moore, T. M., Klein, J. P., Patzakis, M. J. and Harvey, J. P. (1985) Results of compression plating of closed Galeazzi fractures. *Journal of Bone and Joint Surgery,* **67A**, 1015–1021

Table 25.1

Injury	Galeazzi fracture dislocation
Structural impairment	Malunion/imperfect reduction – 90% in conservatively managed
Subjective impairment	Restricted forearm rotation Restricted radiocarpal movement
Disability and handicap	Manual workers handicapped in using tools, skilled craftsmen even more handicapped when using precision instruments Personal toilet and daily living affected
Comments	ORIF of the radial fracture gives 90–100% satisfactory result, but some loss of grip strength is to be expected

26

Fractures of the shaft of the ulna

Isolated fractures of the shaft of the ulna have an unjustified reputation for non-union. In fact the non-union rate is less than 5%. The average time to union in Sarmiento's series was 10 weeks and he reported no cases of non-union (Sarmiento *et al.*, 1976). In contrast, open reduction and internal fixation, while producing excellent functional results, can delay union to over 16 weeks (Burwell and Charnley, 1964). A non-union rate of over 17% has been reported following operative treatment (Brackenbury, Corea and Blakemore, 1981).

References

Brackenbury, P. H., Corea, J. R. and Blakemore, M. E. (1981) Non-union of the isolated fracture of the ulnar shaft in adults. *Injury,* **12**, 371–375

Burwell, H. N. and Charnley, A. D. (1964) Treatment of forearm fractures in adults with particular reference to plate fixation. *Journal of Bone and Joint Surgery,* **46B**, 404–425

Sarmiento, A., Kinman, P. B., Murphy, R. B. and Phillips, J. G. (1976) Treatment of ulnar fractures by functional bracing. *Journal of Bone and Joint Surgery,* **58A**, 1104–1107

Table 26.1

Injury	Fractures of the shaft of the ulna
Structural impairment	Non-union – 5%
Subjective impairment	
Disability and handicap	No disability in 90–95% of patients
Comments	This fracture used to have a (unjustified) reputation for non-union, but open reduction and internal fixation have a higher incidence of delayed and non-union (15% against 5%)

27

Fractures of both bones of the forearm in children

The ability of the growing skeleton to remodel a malunited fracture is nowhere illustrated better than in fractures of the distal radius and ulna. No matter how severe the displacement of the untied fracture, normal anatomy and function is restored within 3 years. Midshaft fractures fare less well. In children under the age of 5 years, complete correction will occur. Over that age the ability to remodel diminishes as puberty approaches. Over the age of 11 years little if any correction is possible (Fuller and McCullough, 1982). Residual angulation of no more than 10° in midshaft fractures of the radius, ulna or both bones, will not restrict rotation of the forearm. Over 20° of residual angulation causes increasing restriction (Matthews *et al.*, 1982).

References

Fuller, D. J. and McCullough, C. J. (1982) Malunited fractures of the forearm in children. *Journal of Bone and Joint Surgery,* **64B**, 364–367

Matthews, L. S., Kaufer, H., Garver, D. F. and Sonstegard, D. A. (1982) The effect on supination-pronation of angular malalignment of both bones of forearm. *Journal of Bone and Joint Surgery,* **64A**, 14–17

Table 27.1

Injury	Fractures of both bones of the forearm in children
Structural impairment	Remodelling potential diminishes with age and distance of fractures from epiphysis *Fractures of distal one third* – complete remodelling in 95% of cases *Fracture of diaphysis* – remodelling, 1–5 years 100%; 6–10 years 50%; 11–14 years 0% } within 3 years
Subjective impairment	A residual angle of 10° in midshaft fractures of radius and ulna will not limit forearm rotation. Loss of movement can be expected with a residual angle of 20° or more
Disability and handicap	Proportionate to restriction of movement
Comments	The only fractures of the lower radius and ulna which did not remodel in Fuller and McCullough's series were in a child aged 14 years

28

Colles' fracture

This most common of fractures has been reviewed extensively. There is agreement that the conventional treatment of reduction and immobilization in a below-elbow plaster cast for 5 weeks results in a high proportion of patients having the residual deformity of a prominent ulnar styloid and dorsal angulation of the lower radius. It has been suggested, and denied, that this malunion constitutes an unacceptable disability. It is agreed that nearly all undisplaced fractures do well.

Controversy arises over the management of displaced fractures; whether treatment should aim for union in anatomical position, and whether residual function is dependent on such position. There is no simple answer, because Colles' fracture is a term used to describe a wide range of injuries, in patients of different ages with different demands on their wrists.

Colles himself wrote that even in the unreduced fracture, full painless movement would return 'at some remote period' (Colles, 1814). This view was supported by Smaill (1965), and, by implication, by many others (Pool, 1973; McAuliffe *et al.,* 1987; Dias *et al.,* 1987). Study of their papers shows that they were mainly concerned with elderly patients, in whom a policy of *laissez faire* seems justified (McQueen, Maclaren and Chalmers, 1986). In the younger patient the restrictions imposed by a malunited Colles' fracture may not be acceptable (Fernandez, 1982), and there is a tendency now to achieve and maintain anatomical reduction (Cooney, Linscheid and Dobyns, 1979).

The complications of Colles' fracture are well known. They occur overall in over 30% of patients (Cooney, Dobyns and Linscheid, 1980). They include malunion, neuropathies, osteoarthrosis of the wrist joint, tendon ruptures, and algodystrophy.

Subjective complaints include pain, limited movement of wrist, forearm and fingers, and weakness of grip. These are due to algodystrophy in a higher number of patients than is realized

(Atkins, Duckworth and Kanis, 1990). Shoulder stiffness in the elderly, rarely mentioned in the literature, is a potential problem.

Overall the results are better in undisplaced fractures with over 90% satisfactory. The elderly have poorer objective results but fewer complaints. Attempts have been made to find radiographic indicators of a poor result. Shortening of the radius 1 week after manipulative reduction appears to be the only consistent sign indicative of a poor functional end result (Villar *et al.*, 1987).

References

Atkins, R. M., Duckworth, T. and Kanis, J. A. (1990) Features of algodystrophy after Colles' fracture. *Journal of Bone and Joint Surgery,* **72B**, 105–110

Colles, A. (1814) On the fracture of the carpal extremity of the radius. *Edinburgh Medical and Surgical Journal,* **10**, 182–186

Cooney, W. P., Dobyns, J. H. and Linscheid, R. L. (1980) Complications of Colles' fracture. *Journal of Bone and Joint Surgery,* **62A**, 613–619

Cooney, W. P., Linscheid, R. L. and Dobyns, J. H. (1979) External pina fixation for unstable Colles' fracture. *Journal of Bone and Joint Surgery,* **61A**, 840–845

Dias, J. J., Wray, C. C., Jones, J. M. and Gregg, P. J. (1987) The value of early mobilisation in the treatment of Colles' fracture. *Journal of Bone and Joint Surgery,* **69B**, 463–467

Fernandez, D. L. (1982) Correction of post-traumatic wrist deformity in adults. *Journal of Bone and Joint Surgery,* **64A**, 1164–1178

McAuliffe, T. B., Hilliar, K. M., Coates, C. J. and Grange, W. J. (1987) Early mobilization of Colles' fracture. *Journal of Bone and Joint Surgery,* **69B**, 727–729

McQueen, M. M., Maclaren, A. and Chalmers, J. (1986) The value of remanipulating Colles' fractures. *Journal of Bone and Joint Surgery,* **68B**, 232–233

Pool, C. (1973) Colles' fracture. *Journal of Bone and Joint Surgery,* **55B**, 540–544

Smaill, G. B. (1965) Long term follow up of Colles' fracture. *Journal of Bone and Joint Surgery,* **47B**, 80–85

Villar, R. N., Marsh, D., Rushton, N. and Greatorex, R. A. (1987) Three years after Colles' fracture. *Journal of Bone and Joint Surgery,* **69B**, 635–638

Table 28.1

Injury	Colles' fracture
Structural impairment	Undisplaced – Little impairment with 90–100% satisfactory results Displaced – Malunion 25–80% – Osteoarthrosis of wrist 3–18% Overall 31% – Median nerve neuropathy 2.5% – Rupture of extensor pollicis longus (EPL) 0.5–1.0% (not associated with displacement)
Subjective impairment	Pain – 75% Restricted movement – almost universal in displaced fractures Weakness of grip – 30–40% Subjective symptoms do not correlate with the cosmetic result, particularly in the elderly
Disability and handicap	The elderly patient may tolerate persistent deformity with weakness of grip, and suffer no handicap. The disability constitutes a positive handicap in those engaged in heavy manual work or who require a normal range of wrist movements, such as muscians, craftsmen, mechanics and surgeons
Comments	Pain and stiffness due to algodystrophy, or Sudeck's atrophy, is more common than is realized, occurring in 37% of cases. The symptoms are often mild and short lived

29

Anterior displacement of the lower radius: Smith's and Barton's fractures

Much less common than Colles' fractures, Smith's and Barton's fractures are similar in that redisplacement of the lower fragment is likely to occur after reduction, and in that residual disability is slight (Thompson and Grant, 1977). Brian Thomas showed that holding the forearm in supination, and the wrist in flexion, confers stability on the reduced fracture (Thomas, 1957). Internal fixation has been advised (Ellis, 1965). The incidence of post-traumatic osteoarthrosis of the wrist joint after Barton's fracture has been reported as 12.5% (De Oliveira, 1973).

References

De Oliveira, J. C. (1973) Barton's fractures. *Journal of Bone and Joint Surgery*, **55A**, 586–594

Ellis, J. (1965) Smith's and Barton's fractures. *Journal of Bone and Joint Surgery*, **47B**, 724–727

Thomas, F. B. (1957) Reduction of Smith's fracture. *Journal of Bone and Joint Surgery*, **39B**, 463–470

Thompson, G. H. and Grant, T. T. (1977) Barton's fractures – reverse Barton's fractures. *Clinical Orthopaedics*, **122**, 210–221

Table 29.1

Injury	Anterior displacement of the lower radius: Smith's and Barton's fractures
Structural impairment	Malunion – 70% after conservative management, 14% after Thomas' manoeuvre Osteoarthrosis of wrist joint – 12%
Subjective impairment	Restricted pronation in less than 10% if fracture is splinted in supination
Disability and handicap	Minimal even with malunion
Comments	

30

Displacement of the lower radial epiphysis

The majority of these injuries are of the Salter/Harris II type where a tongue of metaphysis is displaced with the epiphysis (Salter and Harris, 1963). Precise reduction is not necessary, remodelling is usually total and there is no residual disability. Premature fusion is rare. It can follow over-enthusiastic attempts to obtain anatomical reduction. If the fusion is eccentric, overgrowth deformity can result (Aitken, 1935; Lee, Esterhai and Das, 1984).

References

Aitken, A. P. (1935) The end results of the fractured distal radial epiphysis. *Journal of Bone and Joint Surgery,* **17**, 302–308

Lee, B. S., Esterhai, J. L. and Das, M. (1984) Fracture of the distal radial epiphysis. *Clinical Orthopaedics,* **185**, 90–96

Salter, R. B. and Harris, W. R. (1963) Injuries involving the epiphyseal plate. *Journal of Bone and Joint Surgery,* **45A**, 587–622

Table 30.1

Injury	Separation of the lower radial epiphysis
Structural impairment	Majority are Salter/Harris Type II, with Salter/Harris Type I being next in frequency Premature fusion of the epiphysis in 7% overall
Subjective impairment	
Disability and handicap	Remodelling is almost always complete and anatomical reduction is not necessary. There is no residual disability except when partial premature fusion occurs to be followed by overgrowth deformity
Comments	

31

Fractures of the scaphoid

Fractures of the carpal scaphoid are seen most frequently in men of working age. The length of treatment often necessary to achieve bony union has significant economic implications in such patients, and recent papers have challenged the policy of prolonged conservative treatment (Herbert and Fisher, 1984).

The complications of a fractured scaphoid are delayed union, avascular necrosis, non-union, carpal instability and osteoarthrosis. The complications are affected by the violence of the original injury, the site and type of fracture and the time of diagnosis.

Avascular necrosis is seen in up to 40% of fractures of the proximal third. Union may not occur in these fractures for up to 14 weeks.

Instability of the carpus, shown by separation of the fragments, is associated with non-union and osteoarthrosis (Fisk, 1970; Leslie and Dickson, 1981).

Fractures of the tubercle almost always unite, those more proximally in over 90% of cases. Fractures through the waist, produced by severe violence and with separation of the fragments, are the most prone to non-union. It has been suggested that the rate of non-union in these injuries is as high as 50% (Herbert and Fisher, 1984).

Non-union results in the progressive development of cystic changes in the scaphoid and osteoarthrosis of the wrist. The incidence of degenerative change reaches 100% after 10 years (Mack *et al.*, 1984).

Prompt diagnosis and immediate immobilization are said to diminish the risk of non-union. The policy of diagnosing on suspicion, immobilizing in plaster and repeating the X-rays in 2 weeks was laid down by Watson-Jones (1955) and is followed in most British hospitals to this day. The value of repeat X-rays has been questioned (Dias *et al.*, 1990). Features of poor prognostic import have been identified as: a history of severe direct injury;

separation of the fragments; increasing visibility of the fracture line; early appearance of cystic change (Leslie and Dickson, 1981).

Non-union in itself, or associated with osteoarthrosis of the wrist, is not necessarily a cause of symptoms (London, 1961). Symptoms may only become manifest after a further injury, when radiography reveals long-standing degenerative changes associated with an old ununited scaphoid fracture (Watson-Jones, 1955). A recent paper has shown that even orthopaedic surgeons can remain unaware of this fracture (Brenkel, Pearse and Gregg, 1986).

References

Brenkel, I. J., Pearse, M. and Gregg, P. J. (1986) A 'cracking' complication of haemiarthroplasty of the hip. *British Medical Journal,* **293**, 1648

Dias, J. J., Thompson, J., Barton, N. and Gregg, P. J. (1990) Suspected scaphoid fractures. *Journal of Bone and Joint Surgery,* **72B**, 98–101

Fisk, G. R. (1970) Carpal instability of the fractured scaphoid. *Annals of the Royal College of Surgeons England,* **46**, 63–76

Herbert, T. J. and Fisher, W. E. (1984) Management of the fractured scaphoid using a new bone screw. *Journal of Bone and Joint Surgery,* **66B**, 114–123

Leslie, J. J. and Dickson, R. A. (1981) The fractured carpal scaphoid. *Journal of Bone and Joint Surgery,* **63B**, 225–230

London, P. S. (1961) The broken scaphoid bone. *Journal of Bone and Joint Surgery,* **43B**, 237–244

Mack, G. R., Bosse, M. J., Gelberman, R. H. and Yu, E. (1984) The natural history of scaphoid non-union. *Journal of Bone and Joint Surgery,* **66A**, 504–509

Watson-Jones, R. (1955) *Fractures and Joint Injuries*, 4th edn, Vol. II, E. & S. Livingstone, Edinburgh and London, pp. 606–620

Table 31.1

Injury	Fractures of the scaphoid
Structural impairment	Delayed union – waist fractures may not unite for 14–16 weeks Non-union – 5% Avascular necrosis – up to 40% in proximal third fractures Osteoarthrosis – 100% after 10 years of non-union
Subjective impairment	Pain Weakness of grip Symptoms do not correlate with the radiographic appearances of non-union or degenerative change
Disability and handicap	The fracture occurs predominantly in young men, who also have the highest incidence of displaced fractures through the waist which take longer to unite and have most non-unions. Two to three months away from work is to be expected
Comments	

32

Fractures, dislocations and fracture dislocations of the carpus

Isolated fractures of every carpal bone have been described. A bewildering variety of carpal dislocations, with or without fracture, centre on the lunate; and the whole carpus can dislocate on the radius but this is extremely rare. As one would expect, good results depend on accurate reduction being maintained until bony and ligamentous healing has occurred.

There is a high incidence of malunion, non-union and late degenerative change. Median nerve lesions are common (Campbell, Lance and Yeoh, 1964; Green and O'Brien, 1979; Rawlings, 1981; Adkinson and Chapman, 1982; Moneim, Hofammann and Omer, 1984).

References

Adkinson, J. W. and Chapman, M. W. (1982) Treatment of acute lunate and perilunate dislocations. *Clinical Orthopaedics,* **164**, 199–207

Campbell, R. D., Lance, E. M. and Yeoh, C. B. (1964) Lunate and perilunar dislocations. *Journal of Bone and Joint Surgery,* **46B**, 55–72

Green, D. P. and O'Brien, E. T. (1979) Classification and management of carpal dislocations. *Clinical Orthopaedics,* **149**, 55–72

Moneim, M. S., Hofammann, K. E. and Omer, G. E. (1984) Trans-scaphoid perilunate fracture-dislocation. *Clinical Orthopaedics,* **190**, 227–235

Rawlings, D. (1981) The management of dislocations of the carpal lunate. *Injury,* **12**, 319–330

Table 32.1

Injury	Fractures, dislocations and fracture dislocations of the carpus
Structural impairment	Malunion/malalignment – 40–70% Non-union – (of scaphoid) up to 75% Osteoarthrosis – Over 50% Median nerve lesion – 30–60%. Neurapraxia.
Subjective impairment	Pain – 60% Stiffness – Loss of 50% wrist movement almost inevitable Weakness of grip – 40%
Disability and handicap	Manual workers significantly handicapped after the more serious injuries. Average time lost from work 6 months – 1 year
Comments	

33
Hand injuries

In this section, injuries of particular structures are dealt with individually. In practice, matters are not so simple. Many injuries may exist together and the prognosis for hand function becomes correspondingly more difficult. Complications such as loss of skin and infection have an effect on the end result. Crush injuries are slower to heal than 'sharp' injuries, with swelling and tissue necrosis delaying the return of movement. Prolonged attempts at reconstruction may worsen prognosis; in an unskilled worker selective amputation may allow return to work sooner and with less residual disability (London, 1961).

Reference

London, P. S. (1961) Simplicity of approach to the injured hand. *Journal of Bone and Joint Surgery,* **43B**, 454–464

Fractures of the metacarpals

The most common metacarpal fracture is that of the neck of the fifth. Some degree of malunion is usual, with depression of the knuckle. Unless the residual angulation is gross, the functional disability is negligible as finger movement is not impeded. The cosmetic blemish is apparent when the fist is clenched.

Fractures of the base of the first metacarpal involving the carpometacarpal joint (Bennett's fracture) will, like all intra-articular fractures, result in limited movement of the joint unless accurate reduction is achieved and maintained (Pollen, 1968). There is a 12.5% incidence of post-traumatic osteoarthrosis of the carpometacarpal joint in imperfectly reduced fractures (Griffiths, 1964). The loss of movement produces little disability. In Griffiths' series of 21 cases, eight patients had residual symptoms. Of these, seven were assessed as trivial and only one as marked (Griffiths, 1964). In an attempt to find a relationship between Bennett's fracture and later osteoarthrosis, Griffiths (1964) reviewed 46 cases of carpometacarpal osteoarthrosis who presented for treatment. In none of them did he find evidence of old fracture.

References

Griffiths, J. C. (1964) Fractures at the base of the first metacarpal bone. *Journal of Bone and Joint Surgery,* **46B**, 712–719

Pollen, A. G. (1968) The conservative treatment of Bennetts fracture-subluxation of the first metacarpal. *Journal of Bone and Joint Surgery,* **50B**, 91–101

Table 33.1

Injury	Fractures of the base of the first metacarpal
Structural impairment	Malunion – varus deformity at base of metacarpal Osteoarthrosis of carpometacarpal joint 12.5%
Subjective impairment	Pain on gripping Weakness of grip Limited thumb movement } symptoms trivial in 97.5%
Disability and handicap	Significant disability is rare
Comments	The results of imperfect reduction produce such little residual disability in the long term that it is doubtful whether operative fixation of Bennett's fracture is justified

Fractures of the fingers

Malunion of fractured phalanges, producing rotational or angulated deformity, can inflict significant disability on the patient. Intra-articular fractures involving the interphalangeal joints can cause residual pain and stiffness. Inability to close the fingers to the palm constitutes a disability and a handicap in manual workers (Barton, 1977).

Reference

Barton, N. (1977) Fractures of the phalanges of the hand. *Hand,* **9**, 1–10

Table 33.2

Injury	Fractures of the phalanges
Structural impairment	Malunion – angulatory or rotational – intra-articular
Subjective impairment	Inability to bring finger tip to palm Impaired grip
Disability and handicap	Restricted ability to perform fine movments Handicap in manual workers and craftsmen
Comments	

Tendon injuries in the hand

The terminal slip of the extensor tendon proximal to, or at the level of, the terminal interphalangeal (TIP) joint may be ruptured by indirect trauma, producing a mallet finger. Other extensor tendon divisions are produced by incised wounds. The disability from a mallet finger is trivial although the lesion can be painful for some months. Division of the central slip of the tendon proximal to the proximal interphalangeal (PIP) joint produces an increasing deformity of flexion at the proximal interphalangeal level with hyperextension at the terminal joint (the bouttoniere deformity). The deformity is ugly but the resulting disability is a handicap only to skilled manual workers or artists. Repairs of the main extensor tendon do well, apart from a tendency to adherence. This may result in some loss of finger flexion.

Flexor tendon injuries are another matter altogether. Inability to bend a finger, particularly to oppose it to the thumb, is a considerable disability. A stiff extended finger is a nuisance. The results of flexor tendon repair have improved steadily of recent years with the improvement in the training of hand surgeons, the growth of microsurgery and the increased availability of hand surgery centres. Even so, the results of flexor tendon repair in the 'no mans land' of the hand, between the distal palmar crease and the middle of the finger, are, at best, 80% successful (Strickland and Glogovac, 1980; Amadio and Hunter, 1987). In regions proximal and distal to this middle zone, the results of repair, particularly if carried out early, are much better (Lister, Kleiners and Kutz, 1977).

References

Amadio, P. C. and Hunter, J. M. (1987) Prognostic factor in flexor tendon surgery in zone 2. In *Tendon Surgery in the Hand* (eds J. M. Hunter, L. H. Schneider and E. J. Machin), C. V. Mosby, St. Louis, pp. 138–147

Lister, G. D., Kleiners, H. E. and Kutz, J. E. (1977) Primary flexor tendon repair. *Journal of Hand Surgery*, **2**, 441–451

Strickland, J. W. and Glogovac, S. C. (1980) Digital function following flexor tendon repair in zone 2. *Journal of Hand Surgery*, **5**, 537

Table 33.3

Injury	Extensor tendon division in the hand
Structural impairment / **Subjective impairment**	At metacarpophalangeal (MCP) level – inability to extend MCP joint At proximal interphalangeal level (central slip) – inability to extend PIP joint, hyperextension at TIP joint (bouttoniere deformity) At distal interphalangeal joint – inability to extend TIP join (mallet finger)
Disability and handicap	Disability of bouttoniere and mallet lesions diminishes with time as adaptation occurs
Comments	Results of extensor tendon repair at MCP level good but may be slight lag to extension. Bouttoniere lesions are best dealt with soon after injury but the diagnosis is often missed

Table 33.4

Injury	Flexor tendon division in the hand
Structural impairment / **Subjective impairment**	Complete loss of finger flexion if both tendons divided Loss of tip flexion if profundus only divided
Disability and handicap	
Comments	Results of repair vary with level of division and skill of surgeon. In zone 2 results vary from 50% satisfactory to 80% excellent in specialized hand centres. Best results follow primary repair

Industrial injection injuries of the hand

These are uncommon injuries but with a poor prognosis unless recognized and treated promptly. If neglected, extensive tissue necrosis, infection and scarring will follow leaving a stiff, useless digit which usually requires amputation. The materials injected have included oil, grease (Sharrard, 1968), paint (Stark, Ashworth and Boyes, 1967) and cement (Hutchinson, 1968).

References

Hutchinson, C. H. (1968) Hand injuries caused by injection of cement under pressure. *Journal of Bone and Joint Surgery,* **50B**, 131–133

Sharrard, W. J. W. (1968) Industrial injection injuries. *Journal of Bone and Joint Surgery,* **50B**, 1

Stark, H., Ashworth, C. R. and Boyes, J. H. (1967) Paintgun injuries of the hand. *Journal of Bone and Joint Surgery,* **49A**, 637–641

Table 33.5

Injury	Industrial injection injuries of the hand
Structural impairment	Tissue necrosis, Infection } Fibrosis → stiffness
Subjective impairment	
Disability and handicap	The disability of a stiff digit may necessitate amputation
Comments	Prognosis depends on prompt recognition and treatment Recovery is prolonged even in those treated early

Vibration white finger

Recently accepted as an industrial disease in the United Kingdom, this condition affects workers using powered vibration tools such as chainsaws and drills. Its aetiology is unknown but it needs to be distinguished from Raynaud's phenomenon. The long-term prognosis is uncertain as yet but sufferers are advised to avoid handling vibration tools out of doors (Boyle, Smith and Burke, 1988).

Reference

Boyle, J. C., Smith, N. J. and Burke, F. D. (1988) Vibration white finger. *Journal of Hand Surgery,* **13B**, 171–176

Table 33.6

Injury	Vibration white finger
Structural impairment	Digital vessel spasm Carpal tunnel syndrome Carpal cysts
Subjective impairment	Pain, numbness, tingling in fingers Finger pallor in cold and when using vibration tools
Disability and handicap	Peculiar to workers using vibrating tools, in forestry, quarry workers, road workers, foundrymen, etc.
Comments	The condition is progressive but can probably be arrested if occupation is changed

34

Overuse syndromes in the upper limb

This group of conditions includes well-defined clinical entities, some of which are recognized as industrial injuries (Prescribed Disease No. A.34; DHSS classification), some which are not. The term Repetitive Stress Syndromes is used as a blanket description for the group (Semple, 1986). Other terms used are Over Use Syndrome, Focal Dystonia, even Conversion Hysteria (Fry, 1986). This section will be confined to those conditions whose origin in excessive hand and wrist activity is not in doubt.

References

Fry, H. J. H. (1986) Overuse syndrome, alias tenosynovitis/tendinitis: the terminological hoax. *Plastic and Reconstructive Surgery,* **78**, 414–417

Semple, C. (1986) Tenosynovitis. *Journal of Hand Surgery,* **11B**, 155–156

Tenosynovitis, peritendinitis crepitans and tenovaginitis

These conditions are recognized in the United Kingdom as Prescribed Disease No.A.34, and industrial compensation is granted. The short-term prognosis is good, as avoidance of the stress responsible brings rapid relief. There is a strong tendency to relapse, particularly on resumption of the causative movement, but the long-term prognosis is good (Thompson, Plewes and Shaw, 1951). Operative decompression may be necessary in de Quervains disease.

Reference

Thompson, A. R., Plewes, L. W. and Shaw, E. G. (1951) Peritendinitis crepitans and simple tenosynovitis. *British Journal of Industrial Medicine,* **8**, 150–155

Table 34.1

Injury	Tenosynovitis and allied conditions
Structural impairment	Inflammatory signs Stenosis of tendon sheaths
Subjective impairment	Pain Swelling
Disability and handicap	Handicap in occupations involving repetitive forearm and wrist movements
Comments	Relapse rate up to 80% Recognized Disease A.34

Traumatic enthesiopathy: lateral and medial epicondylitis

The traumatic origin of these lesions is rarely clear cut, following a single identifiable injury. They are more often associated with repetitive strain although not recognized as industrial injury in the UK.

The overall prognosis in tennis elbow is good, with up to 90% of cases resolving spontaneously. Relapse is common, both after spontaneous resolution and successful treatment (Coonrad and Hooper, 1973). About 3–5% become recalcitrant to non-operative treatment. The failure rate after operative decompression is between 20 and 30% (Limbers, 1980). Fortunately, medial epicondylitis is much less common than the lateral lesion, as in my experience the results of treatment are disappointing.

References

Coonrad, R. W. and Hooper, W. R. (1973) Tennis elbow; its course, natural history, conservative and surgical management. *Journal of Bone and Joint Surgery,* **55A**, 1177–1182

Limbers, P. A. (1980) Tennis elbow. *Journal of Bone and Joint Surgery,* **62B**, 262

Table 34.2

Injury	Tennis elbow: traumatic enthesiopathy
Structural impairment	
Subjective impairment	Pain around outer side of elbow and upper forearm on wrist and hand movement, particularly gripping
Disability and handicap	Pain can interfere with repetitive manual tasks and with gripping working tools or sports equipment
Comments	90% Resolve spontaneously. Residue can be resistant to all forms of treatment

Part 3

The lower limb

35

Dislocations of the hip

Posterior dislocation of the hip joint is an injury produced by severe violence. Simple dislocations, without fractures of the acetabulum and uncomplicated by avascular necrosis of the femoral head, have a 26% chance of developing osteoarthrosis of the hip (Upadhyay and Moulton, 1981). Dislocations associated with fractures of the acetabulum have a worse prognosis, the incidence of complications increasing with the severity of the associated fracture, itself an indicator of the violence of the initial injury. Delay in the reduction of the dislocation has an adverse effect on prognosis.

Avascular necrosis of the femoral head may take 2 years to become radiographically apparent and osteoarthrosis may not become manifest for 5 years. Early prognosis must therefore be provisional. Of the published results of large series, Upadhyay and Moulton's paper is the most useful as it is based on a 12-year follow up and shows that even simple dislocations, quickly reduced, have a significant incidence of residual disability.

Thompson and Epstein (1951) described five subgroups, depending on the site and degree of acetabular fracture. Prognosis of each subgroup is unnecessarily complicated and for practical purposes it suffices to describe simple dislocations and fracture dislocations. Detailed subdivisions of fracture types are never as precise as they first appear and different observers confronted with the same radiograph often disagree about appearances.

References

Thompson, V. P. and Epstein, H. C. (1951) Traumatic dislocation of the hip. *Journal of Bone and Joint Surgery,* **33A**, 746–777

Upadhyay, S. S. and Moulton, A. (1981) The long term results of traumatic posterior dislocation of the hip. *Journal of Bone and Joint Surgery,* **63B**, 548–551

Table 35.1

Injury	Posterior dislocation of the hip without fracture
Structural impairment	Avascular necrosis of the femoral head 16%. May take 2 years to become apparent Osteoarthrosis of the hip joint 26%. May not become symptomatic for 5 years
Subjective impairment	Pain Stiffness Deformity
Disability and handicap	That of an osteoarthrotic hip
Comments	Delay in reduction has an adverse effect on prognosis. The risk of avascular necrosis rises to 56% if reduction is delayed longer than 6 hours

Table 35.2

Injury	Posterior fracture dislocation of the hip
Structural impairment	Avascular necrosis of the femoral head 25–70%. May take 2 years to develop Osteoarthrosis of the hip joint 50–75%. May not become symptomatic for 5 years Sciatic nerve palsy <5%
Subjective impairment	Pain Stiffness Limp
Disability and handicap	That of an osteoarthrotic hip
Comments	The wide range of % incidence of complications encompasses the degrees of severity of acetabular fractures. Symptoms will appear earlier in those patients with more extensive fractures

36

Central fracture dislocation of the hip

Post-traumatic osteoarthrosis of the hip occurs in nearly 50% of all fractures of the acetabulum, but the incidence varies considerably between undisplaced fractures and those which produce comminuted displacement of the acetabular roof. Where there is residual displacement, the incidence can be as high as 85%; where there is none, the incidence falls to 30% (Pennal *et al.*, 1980; Mayo, 1987; Tile, Kellam and Joyce, 1985). The immediate clinical result in those with residual displacement of less than 3 mm is good, but a long-term incidence of osteoarthrosis approaching 30% shows that, even in those with an apparently excellent result, the prognosis for hip function is fair only. The more nihilistic among orthopaedic surgeons believe that the main reason for attempting reduction of these complex injuries is to provide optimum conditions for the almost inevitable hip replacement!

Avascular necrosis of the femoral head and myositis ossificans are further, uncommon, complications.

The fracture takes a long time to consolidate but it has been shown that the result 1 year after injury gives a firm indication for the future. Of those patients who show a good result 1 year after injury, 90% will do well. Of those who will develop osteoarthrosis or avascular necrosis of the femoral head, 90% will show evidence of early change at 1 year (Rowe and Lowell, 1961).

A more optimistic picture was drawn by Austin (1971). He reported that 80% of his patients (he reviewed 25 cases) returned to their pre-accident occupation, but nearly half of them had to change or modify their leisure activities. As one would expect, middle-aged and elderly patients fare worse than the young (Tipton, d'Ambrosia and Ryle, 1975).

Other complications of this injury include sciatic nerve paralysis. Tile, Kellam and Joyce (1985) reported a 15% incidence with recovery in only 25% of those affected.

References

Austin, R. T. (1971) Hip function after central fracture dislocation: a long term review. *Injury,* **3**, 114–120

Mayo, K. A. (1987) Fractures of the acetabulum. *Orthopaedic Clinics of North America,* **18**(1), 43–57

Pennal, G. F., Davidson, J., Garside, H. and Plewes, J. (1980) Results of treatment of acetabular fractures. *Clinical Orthopaedics,* **151**, 115–123

Rowe, C. R. and Lowell, D. (1961) Prognosis of fractures of the acetabulum. *Journal of Bone and Joint Surgery,* **434A**, 30–59

Tile, M., Kellam, J. F. and Joyce, M. (1985) Fractures of the acetabulum. *Journal of Bone and Joint Surgery,* **67B**, 324–325

Tipton, W. W., D'Ambrosia, R. D. and Ryle, G. P. (1975) Non-operative management of central fracture dislocation of the hip. *Journal of Bone and Joint Surgery,* **57A**, 888–893

Table 36.1

Injury	Central fracture dislocation of the hip
Structural impairment	Malunion (residual displacement of acetablum) Avascular necrosis of femoral head Osteoarthrosis of hip joint (30–85% depending on residual displacement). Overall 50% Myositis ossificans <5% Sciatic nerve palsy 15%. No recovery in 75%
Subjective impairment	Pain, Stiffness, Limp } with osteoarthrosis. Early clinical results may be excellent or good
Disability and handicap	Up to 80% return to pre-accident occupation Up to 50% have to modify leisure activity
Comments	Prognosis can be firm 1 year after injury Signs of osteoarthrosis and/or avascular necrosis will be apparent then Absence of such signs + good clinical result = good prognosis

37

Fractures of the neck of the femur

Transcervical fractures in the elderly

These fractures may be undisplaced or displaced. The division into Garden's four types is difficult to distinguish in practice and is irrelevant for prognosis (Fransden *et al.*, 1988). Prognosis of the fracture is often secondary to the prognosis for life. The fracture occurs through osteoporotic bone with minimal or no violence and can be one of a sequence of osteoporotic fractures occurring in the other hip, or the spine.

Undisplaced fractures do well with internal fixation; displaced fractures show a high incidence of non-union and avascular necrosis of the femoral head.

Transcervical fractures in the young adult

These fractures occur through healthy bone and are caused by considerable violence. Undisplaced fractures have been reported as showing rates of non-union varying from 0 to 25% and avascular necrosis from 14 to 45%. Displaced fractures fare worse, with non-union of 15–59% and avascular necrosis of 30–85% being described (Protzman and Burkhalter, 1976; Klenerman, 1985).

Trochanteric fractures

Non-union and avascular necrosis are rare in trochanteric fractures but malunion in unstable fractures is common, and is influenced by the method of treatment. When the lesser trochanter is detached, or the fracture is comminuted, union will occur in varus unless rigid internal fixation is applied. Varus deformity will produce a short externally rotated leg.

In the elderly these fractures are associated with a significant mortality rate which is only slightly modified by the form of treatment adopted. Conservative treatment is accompanied by a mortality rate of 30% within 1 year; open reduction and internal fixation is accompanied by a death rate of 16.5% within a similar period (Evans, 1951).

Fractures of the neck of the femur in children

These fractures are sufficiently rare for no single orthopaedic surgeon to have an extensive personal experience. Leung and Lam (1986) and Lam (1971) have reviewed the literature. Long-term reviews are available (Ratliff, 1962; Canale and Bourland, 1977; Leung and Lam, 1986). The injury is the result of severe violence and the prognosis depends on the degree of initial displacement of the fracture. The complications include malunion (coxa vara and premature fusion of the growth plate), non-union and avascular necrosis of the femoral head.

References

Canale, S. T. and Bourland, W. L. (1977) Fractures of the neck and intertrochanteric region of the femur in children. *Journal of Bone and Joint Surgery,* **59A**, 431–443

Evans, E. M. (1951) Trochanteric fractures. *Journal of Bone and Joint Surgery,* **33B**, 192–204

Fransden, P. A., Anderson, E., Madsen, F. and Skjadt, T. (1988) Garden's classification of femoral neck fractures. *Journal of Bone and Joint Surgery,* **70B**, 588–591

Klenerman, L. (1985) The young patient with a fractured neck of femur. *British Medical Journal,* **290**, 1928

Lam, S. F. (1971) Fractures of the neck of the femur in children. *Journal of Bone and Joint Surgery,* **53A**, 1165–1179

Leung, P. C. and Lam, S. F. (1986) Long term follow up of children with femoral neck fractures. *Journal of Bone and Joint Surgery,* **68B**, 537–540

Protzman, R. R. and Burkhalter, M. D. (1976) Femoral neck fractures in young adults. *Journal of Bone and Joint Surgery,* **58A**, 684–694

Ratliff, A. H. C. (1962) Fractures of the neck of the femur in children. *Journal of Bone and Joint Surgery,* **44B**, 528–542

Table 37.1

Injury	Transcervical fractures of the femur in the elderly
Structural impairment	Non-union Avascular necrosis Late segmental collapse } Osteoarthrosis of the hip
Subjective impairment	Pain Stiffness Deformity
Disability and handicap	Loss of independence
Comments	Prognosis in the elderly is dependent on general physical and mental health Avascular necrosis may not become apparent for 2 years

Table 37.2

Injury	Trochanteric fractures in the elderly
Structural impairment	Malunion – varus deformity of neck with shortening and external rotation
Subjective impairment	Limp
Disability and handicap	Impaired walking ability Reliance on walking aids Loss of independence
Comments	These fractures are associated with significant morbidity and mortality

Table 37.3

Injury	Femoral neck fractures in young or middle-aged adults
Structural impairment	Malunion – imperfect reduction contributes to late segmental collapse Non-union – 25% Avascular necrosis – 45% Osteoarthrosis of the hip
Subjective impairment	Pain Stiffness Limp
Disability and handicap	Poor overall results 45% Unable to return to pre-accident employment One review of military personnel showed less than 5% fit to return to pre-accident duty
Comments	

Table 37.4

Injury	Femoral neck fractures in children
Structural impairment	Malunion – coxa vara 54% – premature epiphyseal fusion 54% Non-union – 7% (only in displaced fractures) Avascular necrosis – 36% (91% in displaced fractures)
Subjective impairment	Pain Stiffness –amounting to ankylosis in severe cases (Shortening may be more than 2 cm and may be increased by premature closure of the lower femoral growth plate)
Disability and handicap	Pain and stiffness can severely restrict activity, with surgical intervention necessary
Comments	Avascular necrosis is radiologically apparent within 12 months of injury Symptoms may be delayed until adult life

38

Slipped upper femoral epiphysis

There is an underlying diathesis to this condition, related to hormone imbalance, but presentation may be precipitated by injury. Acute slipping of the epiphysis can follow one episode of injury; more often symptoms of pain and limp precede the injury which precipitates presentation. The condition affects children nearing the end of their growth period and is usually followed by fusion of the epiphysis within 1 year. The time available for growth to remodel any deformity is therefore limited.

The following impairments can ensue:

1. Malunion. The residual deformity is of external rotation, adduction and shortening due to coxa vara. The degree of deformity depends on the severity of the displacement. Coxa vara leads to osteoarthrosis of the hip in adult life.
2. Avascular necrosis of the epiphysis, and, after closure of the growth plate, of the femoral head. Although such necrosis most often follows treatment, that is to say, it is iatrogenic, it is seen rarely in the untreated hip. It occurs within 2 years of the slip and results in a stiff painful hip.
3. Chondrolysis of the femoral articular cartilage is seen in children managed conservatively as well as those treated by operation. Untreated, it causes painful ankylosis of the joint, but there is some evidence that prolonged non-weight-bearing over a 2-year period allows regeneration of the cartilage, and the restoration of normal hip function.

Late diagnosis has an adverse effect on the outcome; without treatment coxa vara is inevitable.

The incidence of bilateral slipping is 65% in the published series, the second hip slipping within a few months after the first, often while the first hip is still under treatment or review.

References

Boyer, D. W., Mickelson, M. R. and Ponseti, J. W. (1981) Slipped capital femoral epiphysis: a long term follow up study of one hundred and twenty patients. *Journal of Bone and Joint Surgery,* **63A**, 85–95

Dunn, D. M. and Angel, J. C. (1978) Replacement of the femoral head by open operation in severe adolescent slipping of the upper femoral epiphysis. *Journal of Bone and Joint Surgery,* **60B**, 394–403

Hall, J. E. (1957) The results of treatment of slipped femoral epiphysis. *Journal of Bone and Joint Surgery,* **39B**, 659–673

Wilson, P. D., Jacobs, B. and Schecter, L. (1965) Slipped capital femoral epiphysis: an end result study. *Journal of Bone and Joint Surgery,* **57A**, 1128–1145

Table 38.1

Injury	Slipped upper femoral epiphysis
Structural impairment	Malunion (coxa vara) Avascular necrosis Chondrolysis
Subjective impairment	Coxa vara may inflict little or no disability but there is a high incidence of osteoarthrosis of the hip in early middle age. Avascular necrosis produces the severe disability of a painful ankylosed hip joint. Chondrolysis may also result in ankylosis. Regeneration may follow prolonged non-weight-bearing
Disability and handicap	A painfully ankylosed hip demands treatment. Arthrodesis of the hip produces a stable, painless joint with surprisingly little handicap even for heavy manual work. Long-term results suggest an increased tendency to low back problems
Comments	The prognosis of promptly diagnosed early slips, treated by pinning *in situ* is excellent with over 90% good results. The outlook is adversely affected by late diagnosis and by the complications of the various operative treatments, concerning which there is much controversy

39

Subtrochanteric fractures of the femur

The short proximal fragment of this fracture tends to be pulled into abduction and flexion by the unopposed action of the abductor and psoas muscles. It is a high velocity injury with extensive soft tissue stripping of the bone ends and an appreciable incidence of non-union. The disappointing results of conservative management has led to a more aggressive approach, with open reduction and internal fixation now being the treatment of choice. The fixator device must be sufficiently robust to overcome the deforming forces, particularly if there has been comminution of the medial femoral cortex, and an intramedullary component to the implant is advisable (Waddell, 1979; Zickel, 1976; Seinsheimer, 1978).

The subtrochanteric area of the femur is a frequent site of pathological fractures.

References

Seinsheimer, F. (1978) Subtrochanteric fractures of the femur. *Journal of Bone and Joint Surgery,* **60A**, 300–306

Waddell, J. P. (1979) Subtrochanteric fractures of the femur. *Journal of Trauma,* **19**, 582–592

Zickel, R. E. (1976) An intramedullary fixation device for the proximal femur. *Journal of Bone and Joint Surgery,* **58A**, 866–872

Table 39.1

Injury	Subtrochanteric fractures of the femur
Structural impairment	Malunion. Varus deformity >10° 46% Shortening >1 inch 14% Non-union 18% Knee stiffness 10% } Overall poor results with conservative treatment 50%
Subjective impairment	The impairment with minor degrees of varus, and shortening of up to 2 cm is minimal Residual deformity greater than this will cause limp Consolidation of union may not occur for 12 months
Disability and handicap	Incapacity for heavy work should be a minimum of 1 year Any residual disability, excepting gross shortening, is not a source of handicap
Comments	The results of internal fixation using an intramedullary device are good, with over 90% good results reported

40

Fractures of the shaft of the femur

This fracture occurs at all ages but is most common in young adults subjected to major violence. It is sometimes associated with other injuries, in the same femur, in the same leg or opposite leg or with multiple injuries. These other injuries complicate management and adversely affect the prognosis of the femoral shaft (Moulton, Upadhyay, Fletcher and Bancroft, 1984). Other injuries in the same leg may reflect the severity of the initial violence and suggest the likelihood of delayed union (Ratcliff, 1968).

It is usually accepted that fractures of the femoral shaft require a year to consolidate (Dencker, 1965). A disturbing rate (4%) of refracture suggests that this is not generally appreciated (Seimon, 1964). Non-union is rare. A degree of malunion, including shortening, is common after conservative treatment and does not cause residual disability unless gross. Up to 2 cm of shortening does not cause a limp.

Knee stiffness reflects the amount of soft tissue damage, or scarring of the quadriceps mechanism (Nichols, 1963). It increases after prolonged immobilization and is associated with delay in union, rather than the choice of treatment (Rokkanen, Slatis and Vankka, 1969).

References

Dencker, H. M. (1965) Shaft fractures of the femur: a comparative study of various methods of treatment in 1003. *Acta Chirurgica Scandinavia,* **130,** 173–184

Moulton, A., Upadhyay, S. S., Fletcher, M. and Bancroft, G. (1984) Does an associated injury affect the outcome of a fracture of the femoral shaft? *Journal of Bone and Joint Surgery,* **66B**, 285

Nichols, P. J. R. (1963) Rehabilitation after fractures of the shaft of the femur. *Journal of Bone and Joint Surgery,* **45B**, 96–102

Ratcliff, A. H. C. (1968) Fractures of the shaft of femur and tibia in the same limb. *Proceedings of the Royal Society of Medicine,* **61**, 906–908

Rokkanen, P., Slatis, P. and Vankka, E. (1969) Closed or open medullary nailing of femoral shaft fractures? A comparison with conservatively treated cases. *Journal of Bone and Joint Surgery,* **51B**, 313–323

Seimon, L. P. (1964) Refracture of the shaft of the femur. *Journal of Bone and Joint Surgery,* **46B**, 32–39

Table 40.1

Injury	Fractures of the shaft of the femur
Structural impairment	Malunion – Shortening 28% with conservative management Varus, Valgus } over 20% Delayed union (including fracture) 4%. Non-union 2% Knee stiffness <90° flexion 17%. < Full flexion 37%
Subjective impairment	
Disability and handicap	Shortening of less than 2 cm is not associated with disability. Angular deformity of less than 10° is not associated with disability. Knee stiffness of less than 100° flexion constitutes a disability. Knee stiffness is the main cause of residual handicap. Less than 100% of flexion interferes with squatting, sitting and climbing stairs. Average time of inability to work 13½ months
Comments	If the fracture is isolated, over 95% of patients can return to their pre-accident occupation. The chances of permanent handicap are increased by the presence of multiple injuries

41

Fractures of the femoral condyles

Experience suggests that the results of this injury are not good and this impression is reinforced by a study of the relevant literature (Laros, 1979; Behrens *et al.*, 1986). Angular deformity, shortening and incongruity of the articular surface of the femur can follow conservative mangement. Osteoarthrosis of the anterior and lateral compartments of the knee is common. In the elderly patient osteoarthrosis may well have been present before the injury. A stiff painful knee with restricted knee movement is common.

Open reduction and accurate internal fixation are claimed to reduce significantly the incidence of post-traumatic osteoarthrosis due to residual incongruity of the joint surface.

References

Behrens, F., Ditmanson, P., Hartleben, P., Comfort, T. H., Gaither, D. W. and Denis, F. (1986) Long term results of distal femoral fractures. *Journal of Bone and Joint Surgery,* **68B**, 848

Laros, G. S. (1979) Supracondylar fractures of the femur. *Clinical Orthopaedics,* **138**, 9–12

Table 41.1

Injury	Fractures of the femoral condyles
Structural impairment	Malunion. Shortening, Angular deformity, Articular surface incongruity – Dependent on management Non-union 5% Osteoarthrosis of knee 25%
Subjective impairment	Overall 66% acceptable results, with no deformity, slight restriction of flexion, and little or no pain Overall incidence of osteoarthrosis 25% Depression of articular surface of more than 3 mm will lead to osteoarthrosis
Disability and handicap	Restrictions imposed on occupations involving standing, climbing, squatting, kneeling
Comments	As with all intra-articular fractures the best results follow anatomical reduction but even with perfect reduction some loss of knee flexion is almost inevitable. The results deteriorate with age

42

Fractures of the lower femoral epiphysis

With 40% of overall growth of the leg occurring at the lower femur it might be expected that fracture separations at the lower femoral growth plate would be followed by a high incidence of leg length discrepancy or angular deformity. The extent and degree of residual deformity depends on the age of the injured child and the remaining capacity for remodelling. The violence of the original trauma is also a guide to the likelihood of later growth disturbance.

A recent review gives an overall incidence of residual angular deformity greater than 5° as 19%, with shortening of more than 2 cm as 24% (Roberts, 1984). The worst prognosis is found in children between the ages of 2 and 11, subjected to severe violence (Riseborough, Barrett and Shapiro, 1983).

The Salter–Harris classification can be used for prognosis, most of these injuries falling into Groups I, II and III. The value of the classification in prognosis has been doubted (Lombardo and Harvey, 1977).

References

Lombardo, S. J. and Harvey, J. P. (1977) Fractures of the distal femoral epiphysis. *Journal of Bone and Joint Surgery,* **59A**, 742–751

Riseborough, E. J., Barrett, I. R. and Shapiro, F. (1983) Growth disturbance following distal femoral epiphyseal fracture separations. *Journal of Bone and Joint Surgery,* **65A**, 885–893

Roberts, J. M. (1984) Fractures and dislocations of the knee. In *Fractures in Children*, Vol. 3 (eds C. A. Rockwood, K. E. Wilkins and R. E. King), J. P. Lippincott, Philadelphia

Table 42.1

Injury	Fractures of the lower femoral epiphysis
Structural impairment	Premature epiphyseal fusion: angular deformity 5° – 19% shortening 2 cm – 24%
Subjective impairment	Knee stiffness 16%
Disability and handicap	No residual disability in 70%
Comments	Residual deformity worst between 2 and 11 year age group

43

Dislocation of the knee

Few orthopaedic surgeons have extensive personal experience of this injury. There have been three cases in the writer's unit in the last 27 years. This tiny series reflects the published results of much larger numbers. One suffered an incomplete peroneal palsy which recovered; one, with an associated displaced fracture of the femoral condyle, was left with a stiff, unstable and painful knee which required arthrodesis; and one did well after closed reduction with an asymptomatic knee joint 9 years later. The published reviews show major vascular or nervous damage in up to 50% of cases (Kennedy, 1963; Meyers and Harvey, 1971). Damage to the popliteal artery may be irreparable and necessitate above-knee amputation (Meyers and Harvey, 1971).

References

Kennedy, J. C. (1963) Complete dislocation of the knee joint. *Journal of Bone and Joint Surgery,* **45A**, 889–903

Meyers, M. H. and Harvey, J. P. (1971) Traumatic dislocation of the knee joint. *Journal of Bone and Joint Surgery,* **53A**, 16–29

Table 43.1

Injury	Dislocation of the knee
Structural impairment	High rate of complications – Popliteal artery damage 16–50% Lateral popliteal nerve injury 33–50%
Subjective impairment	Stiffness, Pain, Instability } of knee
Disability and handicap	Little or no disability 16% Moderate disability 72% Severe disability 12%
Comments	

44

Ruptures of the quadriceps tendon

Sustained by minimal strain, this injury of the elderly is often bilateral and often missed. After operative repair the power of the extensor apparatus to extend the knee is restored but usually at the expense of full flexion. Rerupture has not been recorded.

45

Injuries of the patellar ligament

Avulsion of the ligament from the inferior pole of the patella (Sindig–Larsen–Johannsen disease)

The injury occurs in children and the superficial layers of bony cortex at the origin of the tendon are pulled off the body of the patella, 'like the shell off a hard boiled egg' (Beddow, Corkery and Shatwell, 1963). Union occurs with elongation of the patella. There is no residual functional disability (Houghton and Ackroyd, 1979).

Avulsion of the ligament from the tibial tubercle (Osgood–Schlatter's disease)

The traction apophysis of the upper tibial growth plate is pulled away. Fragmentation may occur. Union results in a permanent bony enlargement of the tibial tubercle. In the overwhelming majority no functional disability remains, but premature fusion of the apophysis with resulting genu recurvatum has been described (Jeffreys, 1965).

Avulsion of the tibial tuberosity

These uncommon injuries occur in adolescents near the end of their growth period and genu recurvatum after reduction has not been reported (Hand, Hand and Dunn, 1971).

References

Beddow, F. H., Corkery, P. H. and Shatwell, G. L. (1963) Avulsion of ligamentum patellae from lower pole of patella. *Journal of the Royal College of Surgeons Edinburgh*, **9**, 66–69

Hand, W. L., Hand, C. R. and Dunn, A. W. (1971) Avulsion fractures of the tibial tubercle. *Journal of Bone and Joint Surgery,* **53A**, 1579–1583

Houghton, G. R. and Ackroyd, C. E. (1979) Sleeve fractures of the patella in children. *Journal of Bone and Joint Surgery,* **61B**, 165–169

Jeffreys, T. E. (1965) Genu recurvatum after Osgood–Schlatters disease. *Journal of Bone and Joint Surgery,* **47B**, 298–301

46

Fractures and dislocations of the patella

The giraffe manages well without a patella, but man is at a disadvantage if his fractured patella is excised, or allowed to unite irregularly. Fractures of the patella are produced by direct or indirect violence, when the extensor mechanism of the knee is disrupted. The prognosis of the two varieties varies.

Fractures produced by direct violence contuse and shatter the articular surface of the patella. There is an incidence of post-traumatic exteoarthrosis of the patellofemoral joint which almost by definition approaches 100%. As usual, the symptoms in the affected individual do not necessarily correlate with the radiographic changes.

The results of excision of the patella for these comminuted fractures are disappointing in the early stages but improve with the passage of time. Quadriceps weakness and a feeling of instability may persist for 2 years or more (Duthie and Hutchinson, 1958). The long-term results are fair with a reported incidence of osteoarthrosis ranging from 0 to 20% (Einola, Aho and Kallio, 1976; Wilkinson, 1977).

Separated transverse fractures treated by open reduction and internal fixation do well if accurate reduction is achieved, but if this is not possible the results are not as good as after excision of the patella (Levack, Flannagan and Hobbs, 1985).

Acute dislocation of the patella is an injury of the adolescent and the young adult. There is an associated incidence of osteochondral fracture of 5%. If the soft tissue lesion is not repaired, there is a 40% chance of recurrent dislocation (Rorabeck and Bobechko, 1976). There may be extra-articular lesions which are responsible for recurrent dislocation (Jeffreys, 1963; Gunn, 1964).

References

Duthie, H. L. and Hutchinson, J. R. (1958) The results of partial and total excision of the patella. *Journal of Bone and Joint Surgery*. **40B**, 75–81

Einola, S., Aho, A. J. and Kallio, P. (1976) Patellectomy after fracture. *Acta Orthopaedica Scandinavia,* **47**, 441–447
Gunn, D. R. (1964) Contraction of the quadriceps muscle. *Journal of Bone and Joint Surgery,* **46B**, 493–497
Jeffreys, T. E. (1963) Recurrent dislocation of the patella due to abnormal insertion of the ilio-tibial tract. *Journal of Bone and Joint Surgery,* **45B**, 740–744
Levack, B., Flannagan, J. P. and Hobbs, S. (1985) Results of surgical treatment of fractures of the patella. *Journal of Bone and Joint Surgery,* **67B**, 416–419
Rorabeck, C. H. and Bobechko, W. P. (1976) Acute dislocation of the patella with osteochondral fracture. *Journal of Bone and Joint Surgery,* **58B**, 237–240
Wilkinson, J. (1977) Fractures of the patella treated by total excision. *Journal of Bone and Joint Surgery,* **59B**, 352–354

Table 46.1

Injury	Fractures of the patella
Structural impairment	Osteoarthrosis – 100% in comminuted fractures Patellectomy – no osteoarthrosis. Calcification in area of excised patella
Subjective impairment	Pain Extensor weakness Instability, particularly on descending stairs } in 39% of patients at 7½-year follow up. Absent in 61% of patients at 7½-year follow up
Disability and handicap	
Comments	The best results in displaced fractures follow accurate reduction and tension band wiring

Table 46.2

Injury	Acute dislocation of patella
Structural impairment	Osteochondral fracture 5% Recurrence of dislocation 40%
Subjective impairment	
Disability and handicap	
Comments	

47

Injuries of the menisci

When a tear of the meniscus is diagnosed the treatment is invariably operative. The range of operative treatment spreads from repair to total menisectomy. Current consensus favours partial menisectomy, either open or arthroscopic.

The long-term prognosis after total menisectomy is poor, with osteoarthrotic change being well nigh inevitable (Fairbank, 1948; Goodfellow, 1980).

Unfortunately, the long-term results after open partial menisectomy are none too encouraging. One review found the late result to be the same whether the menisectomy was partial or total, with only 40% of patients having a normal knee 10 years after operation (Tapper and Hoover, 1969). Other reviews have shown radiographic changes of osteoarthrosis of 60% at 10 years (Gear, 1967) and 75% at 17 years (Johnson *et al.*, 1974).

The short-term results of arthroscopic partial menisectomy are encouraging with over 90% excellent results at 3 years (Dandy and Northmore-Ball, 1981), but so are those of the open operation.

These overall depressing results are partly explained by the frequent association of other injuries in the same knee, reported to be as high as 80% (Noyes *et al.*, 1980).

References

Dandy, D. J. and Northmore-Ball, M. D. (1981) Long term results of arthroscopic partial menisectomy. *Clinical Orthopaedics,* **167**, 34–42

Fairbank, T. J. (1948) Knee joint changes after menisectomy. *Journal of Bone and Joint Surgery,* **30B**, 664–670

Gear, M. W. (1967) The late results of menisectomy. *British Journal of Surgery,* **54**, 270–272

Goodfellow, J. W. (1980) He who hesitates is saved. *Journal of Bone and Joint Surgery,* **62B**, 4–5

Johnson, R. J., Kettelvamp, D. B., Clark, W. and Leaverton, P. (1974) Factors affecting results after menisectomy. *Journal of Bone and Joint Surgery,* **56A**, 719–729

Noyes, F. R., Bassett, R. W., Grood, E. S. and Butler, D. L. (1980) Arthroscopy in acute traumatic haemarthrosis of the knee. *Journal of Bone and Joint Surgery,* **62A**, 687–695

Tapper, E. M. and Hoover, N. W. (1969) Late results after menisectomy. *Journal of Bone and Joint Surgery,* **51A**, 517–526

48

Injuries of the ligaments of the knee

It is customary to describe injuries of knee ligaments as individual lesions, and this is often valid, but prognosis is complicated by the frequent association of other injuries. Rupture of one ligament alone may leave little disability but when accompanied by ruptures of others becomes part of a complex lesion with significant effects on knee function. Perhaps more than in most injuries the disability of an unstable knee only becomes a handicap when the stresses imposed on the joint are beyond those experienced in everyday life, or when they are peculiar to a given occupation. The bank manager who ruptures his anterior cruciate ligament will not be handicapped in the way a steel erector would, but he will be handicapped in his leisure if he is an avid rugby union player.

The diagnosis of knee injuries has become more precise of recent years, with clearer understanding of pathomechanics helped by improved imaging techniques and above all by the arthroscope. The development of sport as an important, highly rewarded professional occupation has also stimulated orthopaedic surgeons in their search for better results.

The ligaments in question are the medial and lateral collateral ligaments, and the joint capsules of which they are condensations, and the cruciate ligaments. For prognosis they will be discussed separately and in combination.

The medial collateral ligament

This may be strained, ruptured alone or in combination with a tear of the medial meniscus and the anterior cruciate ligament (O'Donaghue's triad).

Medial ligament strain is common, associated with a short period of incapacity and has a good prognosis. There is no residual disability and no increased vulnerability to further injury.

Rupture of the medial ligament alone has a good prognosis, with 80–90% good results reported after either conservative treatment or operative repair (Sandberg *et al.*, 1987). Rupture of the medial ligament and capsule accompanied by detachment of the medial meniscus and tearing of the anterior cruciate ligament is a severe injury, yet with good results provided that the meniscus is preserved. Repair of the anterior cruciate does not seem to be necessary to achieve a good result. Hughston and Barrett (1983) reported up to 90% good results, without persisting instability and without osteoarthrotic change, in a 20-year follow up of patients treated by repair of the medial ligament alone. It is interesting, however, that not all of those with such good results chose to return to the sport in which they were injured (only 70% did so).

The lateral ligament complex

Less common than medial ligament ruptures, disruptions of the lateral complex are produced by more severe violence, have a more deleterious effect on knee stability and result in greater residual disability. The unrepaired lesion leaves an unstable and painful knee, but the reported results of reconstructive operations are good, with over 80% of patients able to return to competitive sport (Hughston and Jacobsen, 1985).

The anterior cruciate ligament

Isolated tears of this ligament are uncommon. Rupture is more often accompanied by injury to the medial or lateral capsular complexes. It is well known that patients with long-standing complete anterior cruciate deficiency show positive anterior drawer signs, yet lead active lives with little or no disability arising from their knees. When the accompanying lesion is to the medial side causing anteromedial instability this observation still applies. Reviews by McDaniel and Dameron (1980, 1983) and Grove *et al.* (1983) support this impression. They show that, as long as 18 years after injury, nearly half (46%) of their patients had no pain or instability. Half of the patients reviewed were still playing strenuous games. They also found that radiographic evidence of osteoarthrosis after this long period, although present in over half their cases, was severe only in 5%. They felt that the development of osteoarthrosis was due to menisectomy rather than the cruciate lesion, as the changes were maximal in the medial compartment of the knee.

When the anterior cruciate disruption is complicated by damage to the lateral complex, anterolateral instability, as demonstrated by the pivot shift test, follows. They are rare, but carry a worse prognosis than the anteromedial injuries. A five-year follow up shows fewer than 30% with asymptomatic knees (Satku, Kumar and Ngoi, 1986).

The overall results of all anterior cruciate disruptions show an average of 50% able to return to competitive sport, 40% able to play at a less demanding level or at a different sport – swimming or windsurfing instead of rugby football for example – and 10% having to give up sport altogether.

A high incidence of osteoarthrosis is reported, and is thought to follow menisectomy rather than the cruciate deficiency. Severe osteoarthrosis is reported as being between 2 and 9%.

The cruciate-deficient knee will be apparent on clinical examination even although the functional disability is slight. Residual symptoms, when present, are instability, pain and swelling.

Rupture of the posterior cruciate ligament

These uncommon injuries carry an indifferent prognosis. Residual symptoms of pain are common. Pain is usually associated with exertion. Instability is felt when walking on rough ground, coming down stairs and on squatting. Frankly poor end results, with abandonment of sport, amount to 20% (Dandy and Pusey, 1982). The posterior drawer sign is always positive (Trickey, 1968).

References

Dandy, D. J. and Pusey, R. (1982) Long term results of unrepaired tears of the posterior cruciate ligament. *Journal of Bone and Joint Surgery,* **64B**, 92–94

Grove, T. P., Miller, S. J. and Garrick, J. G. (1983) Non-operative treatment of the anterior cruciate ligament. *Journal of Bone and Joint Surgery,* **65A**, 184–192

Hughston, J. C. and Barrett, G. R. (1983) Acute anteromedial rotatory instability. *Journal of Bone and Joint Surgery,* **65A**, 145–153

Hughston, J. C. and Jacobsen, K. (1985) Chronic posterolateral instability. *Journal of Bone and Joint Surgery,* **67A**, 351–359

McDaniel, W. J. and Dameron, T. B. (1980) Untreated ruptures of the anterior cruciate ligament. *Journal of Bone and Joint Surgery,* **62A**, 669–673

McDaniel, W. J. and Dameron, T. B. (1983) The untreated anterior cruciate ligament rupture. *Clinical Orthopaedics,* **172**, 158–163

Sandberg, R., Balkfors, B., Nilsson, B. and Westlin, N. (1987) Operative versus non-operative treatment of recent injury to the ligaments of the knee. *Journal of Bone and Joint Surgery,* **69A**, 1120–1126

Satku, K., Kumar, V. P. and Ngoi, S. S. (1986) Anterior cruciate ligament, to counsel or to operate. *Journal of Bone and Joint Surgery,* **68B**, 458–461

Trickey, E. L. (1968) Rupture of the posterior cruciate ligament. *Journal of Bone and Joint Surgery,* **50B**, 334–341

Table 48.1

Injury	Rupture of the medial collateral ligament of the knee
Structural impairment	Healing of the isolated lesion, resulting in no instability, occurs in over 80% of patients Late osteoarthrosis (at 20 years) in less than 10%
Subjective impairment	Minimal medial instability
Disability and handicap	70% of patients able to return to competitive sport No significant handicap in daily living
Comments	

Table 48.2

Injury	Rupture of the lateral ligament complex of the knee
Structural impairment	Lateral and posterolateral instability in the untreated case
Subjective impairment	The unrepaired lesion results in a painful, unstable knee giving way into hyperextention
Disability and handicap	Restriction on sporting activities, but symptoms even in everyday activities may require the wearing of a knee splint or brace
Comments	The reported results of operative repair are good, with 80% good results found at two year follow up

Table 48.3

Injury	Rupture of the anterior cruciate ligament
Structural impairment	Anterior cruciate deficiency — With anteromedial instability; With anterolateral instability
Subjective impairment	Instability Pain Swelling
Disability and handicap	Anteromedial 46% no pain or instability. Osteoarthrosis in 5% 50% coninue to play strenuous games Anteromedial >30% fully active at 5 years. Osteoarthrosis in 10%
Comments	Overall results 50% return to competitive sport 40% return to sport at a lower level 10% give up sport altogether Symptomatic osteoarthrosis 10%. Thought to be due to loss of meniscus rather than cruciate instability

Table 48.4

Injury	Rupture of the posterior cruciate ligament
Structural impairment	Posterior cruciate deficiency. Posterior drawer sign. Fixed flexion deformity
Subjective impairment	Instability, Pain, Swelling } on exertion
Disability and handicap	Restricted sporting ability Restricted ability to work on rough ground or at work involving squatting, ladders
Comments	

49

Fractures of the condyles of the tibia

These fractures are intra-articular and their prognosis depends on the degree of residual deformity of the articular surface. When there is no displacement of the fracture, or when accurate reduction has been obtained and held, the outlook is excellent. Even under these circumstances, however, there is a possibility that osteoarthrosis of the knee joint will develop. This was found to be 13% in Rasmusen and Sorensen's (1973) series. Many of these fractures occur in the elderly, in patients already showing radiographic evidence of osteoarthrosis. The injury in these patients will accelerate the arthrotic changes, but cannot have caused them.

Malunion of the depressed fragment will result in deformity of the knee. This deformity results in instability of the joint, either in valgus or varus according to site. Instability produces pain and limp. Porter (1970) found a direct association between the depth of the step in the tibial surface and the end result, with poor results in 80% of those with more than 1.4 cm of depression. Accurate measurement of the depth of the depression depends on the positioning of the X-ray tube. The beam should be set at 115°, to allow for the backwards slope of the articular surface of the tibia (Moore and Harvey, 1974). Apley (1956), however, found no such correlation, or between the radiographic appearances of degenerative changes and the functional result. His review was confined to lateral condylar fractures. Other reviews show correlation between residual instability, osteoarthrosis and a poor functional result. A residual varus deformity caused greater disability than valgus as one would expect, with medial fractures being followed by a 21% incidence of osteoarthrosis against lateral fractures of 16%. When deformity followed varus malalignment the incidence of osteoarthrosis rose to 79%, after valgus 31% (Rasmussen and Sorensen, 1973).

References

Apley, A. G. (1956) Fractures of the lateral tibial condyle. *Journal of Bone and Joint Surgery,* **38B**, 699–706

Hohl, M. and Luck, J. V. (1956) Fractures of the tibial condyle. *Journal of Bone and Joint Surgery,* **38A**, 1001–1018

Moore, T. H. and Harvey, J. P. (1974) Roentgenographic measurement of the tibial depression due to fracture. *Journal of Bone and Joint Surgery,* **56A**, 155–160

Porter, R. B. (1970) Crush fractures of the lateral tibial table. *Journal of Bone and Joint Surgery,* **52B**, 676–687

Rasmussen, P. S. and Sorensen, S. E. (1973) Tibial condylar fractures. *Injury,* **4**, 265

Table 49.1

Injury	Fractures of the tibial condyles
Structural impairment	Malunion from condylar depression producing valgus or varus deformity. Deformity associated with development of osteoarthrosis; 31% in valgus deformity, 80% in varus, but osteoarthrosis followed anatomical alignment in 13% Poor correlation between deformity and functional result, but patients with poor results had a high incidence of osteoarthrosis (89%)
Subjective impairment	Painful instability of knee Stiffness – over 1.4 cm depression = 80% chance of poor result (Porter) – over 1.0 cm depression = 40% chance of poor result (Hohl and Luck) Fatigue – disability unrelated to radiogrpahs (Apley) } Disability related to deformity
Disability and handicap	Inability to work related to instability, stiffness and pain Symptoms may demand the wearing of a splint or the use of a walking stick
Comments	The depth of residual depression is observed at fracture union, and prognosis given then Overall excellent or good results in reviewed series 72%

50

Fractures of the shaft of the tibia

The prognosis of fractures of the tibia depends on the violence of the original injury. Closed undisplaced fractures without comminution unite readily with little or no residual impairment or disability. Open fractures, extensively comminuted and associated with severe soft tissue injury, are slow to unite and easily infected. The end result is marred by stiffness of the ankle and subtalar joints. The results of closed and operative treatment are comparable but it must be remembered that a failed operation can result in catastrophe. There are few worse disasters than that of a simple fracture of the tibia which would unite readily in a plaster cast becoming infected after open reduction and ending in amputation.

Ellis (1958a,b) classified tibial fractures into three grades of severity, ranging from minor to severe. His grades are: I, undisplaced or angulated bony fragments (closed or compound from within); II, displaced or comminuted bony fragments (minor compound wound); III, displaced fragments with major comminution (major compound wound).

Nicoll modified this approach by identifying four features as significant in prognosis. Three of these are the same as Ellis', displacement, comminution and soft tissue damage. He added a fourth, infection. This last, of course, can be a consequence of the injury or may be introduced by treatment (Nicoll, 1964). The complications that can occur in these fractures are outlined below.

1. Malunion. This has been defined as shortening of more than 2 cm (Sarmiento, 1967), or angular deformity of more than 10° varus or valgus. Deformities within these limits result in no disability.
2. Delayed and non-union. The incidence rises with the degree of displacement and the extent of soft tissue damage. Delayed union is accepted as being present when the fracture is mobile at 20 weeks. Some orthopaedic surgeons feel that a shorter

period, say 12–15 weeks, should be used. In this context, it is interesting to notice that in 125 cases of tibial fractures, treated in Uganda by virtually unrestricted weight bearing, the average time to union was 9 weeks. Only one fracture did not unite. The rate and severity of malunion, however, was unacceptably high (de Souza, 1987). It is not possible to use these criteria for periods of delayed union when the fracture has been fixed rigidly.

3. Infection. If present, it has an adverse effect on union, and the final result (Nicoll, 1964).
4. Joint stiffness. Affecting mainly the ankle and subtalar joints, it has been reported as 9% (Nicoll, 1964) to 72% (McMaster, 1976). Subtalar movement of less than half the normal range inflicts a significant disability, and affects a patient's ability to return to work.
5. Ischaemic contracture. This is probably more common than is recognized (Owen and Tsimboukis, 1967), and may be a responsible factor in hindfoot stiffness (J. R. Hughes, personal communication). Ellis (1958a,b) reported it in 4% of his patients.

The results set out in the tables are derived from the reported series of fractures treated by closed methods, with or without early weight bearing (Ellis, 1958a,b; Nicoll, 1964; Sarmiento, 1967). It is against this background that the results of operative treatment must be assessed. Some published reviews show spectacularly better results; but it must be stressed again that the consequences of turning a closed fracture into a compound fracture by operation can lead to disaster. Such operations should only be done by skilled surgeons experienced in the principles and practice of rigid internal fixation (Ruedi, Webb and Allgower, 1976).

Whether the integrity of the fibula affects the speed of union is debatable. The patient's age and level of the fracture do not affect the result (Ellis, 1958a,b; Nicoll, 1964).

Hicks (1964) assessed the results of the treatment of tibial fractures by using the incidence of amputation as an index of success. Of 1400 patients reviewed, 55 came to amputation (3.9%).

Fractures of the shaft of the tibia in children do well with little or no residual disability, provided rotational malunion does not occur (Hansen, Greiff and Bergmann, 1976).

References

de Souza, L. J. (1987) Healing time of tibial fractures in Ugandan Asians. *Journal of Bone and Joint Surgery*, **69B**, 56

Ellis, H. (1958a) The speed of healing after fractures of the tibial shaft. *Journal of Bone and Joint Surgery,* **40B**, 42–46
Ellis, H. (1958b) Disabilities after tibial shaft fractures. *Journal of Bone and Joint Surgery,* **40B**, 190–197
Hansen, B. A., Greiff, J. and Bergmann, F. (1976) Fractures of the tibia in children. *Acta Orthopaedica Scandinavia,* **47**, 448–453
Hicks, J. H. (1964) Amputation in fractures of the tibia. *Journal of Bone and Joint Surgery,* **46B**, 388–392
McMaster, M. (1976) Disability of the hindfoot after fracture of the tibial shaft. *Journal of Bone and Joint Surgery,* **58B**, 90–93
Nicoll, E. A. (1964) Fractures of the tibial shaft. *Journal of Bone and Joint Surgery,* **46B**, 373–387
Owen, R. and Tsimboukis, B. (1967) Ischaemia complicating closed tibial and fibular shaft fractures. *Journal of Bone and Joint Surgery,* **49B**, 268
Ruedi, T., Webb, J. K. and Allgower, M. (1976) Experience with the dynamic compression plate in 418 recent fractures of the tibial shaft. *Injury,* **7**, 252–265
Sarmiento, A. (1967) A functional below-knee cast for tibial fractures. *Journal of Bone and Joint Surgery,* **49A**, 855–875

Table 50.1

Injury	Fractures of the tibia. Ellis Grade I
Structural impairment	Delayed or non-union – 2–9% Malunion – less than 5% Joint stiffness – 1–12% Ischaemic contracture – 4%+
Subjective impairment	Pain – none Limp – none } in over 90%
Disability and handicap	None
Comments	

Table 50.2

Injury	Fractures of the tibia. Ellis Grade II
Structural impairment	Delayed/non-union – 11–35% Malunion – as in Grade I Joint stiffness – 5–20% Ischaemic contracture – as in Grade I
Subjective impairment	Pain – moderate Limp – slight limp
Disability and handicap	Restricted ability to walk on rough/uneven ground Prolonged standing/squatting/kneeling difficult
Comments	

Table 50.3

Injury	Fractures of the tibia. Ellis Grade III
Structural impairment	Delayed/non-union – 40–60% Joint stiffness – up to 60% (overall 72% hindfoot stiffness in McMaster's series)
Subjective impairment	Pain – severe Limp – significant
Disability and handicap	Ability to perform physical work significantly impaired 80% of workers in heavy industry unable to return to pre-accident work
Comments	These results apply to fractures treated conservatively

51

Fractures of the ankle

The different classifications of ankle fractures are valuable for understanding the mechanics of injury and for planning treatment. They contribute to prognosis only insofar as they indicate the severity of the initial injury. The end results of fractures of the ankle are directly proportional to the accuracy of the reduction whether the reduction is achieved by closed or open methods of treatment. If an ankle fracture unites in an anatomical position, there is an 85% change of an excellent or good result (Lindsjo, 1981).

An excellent result is an ankle joint indistinguishable from normal. A good result is a shapely ankle with slight, intermittent pain or swelling. A poor result is a stiff, painful and swollen or deformed ankle.

The possible complications affecting these results are: non-union of the medial malleolus; malunion; osteoarthrosis of the ankle joint.

Non-union of the medial malleolus, due to the interposition of soft tissue, occurs in 20% of patients treated conservatively but only 1% of those treated by open reduction (Lindsjo, 1981). The functional results of non-union have been reported as minimal, causing local discomfort, or as contributory to osteoarthrosis (Mendelsohn, 1965). Personal experience supports the former conclusion.

Malunion varies from severe residual displacement with deformity to degrees of incongruence of the ankle mortice detectable on X-ray. This may be very apparent but subtle malalignment may escape the eye. Sarkisian and Cody (1976) describe the talocrural angle which can be used in prognosis. Lines are drawn along the articular surface of the tibia, and between the tips of the malleoli on a true antero-posterior (AP) film. A perpendicular from the articular line crosses the intermalleolar line at an angle of 83 ± 4°. In normal ankles the angle is virtually identical on either side. A variation of more than 5° is of prognostic significance (Phillips *et al.,* 1985). Malunion predisposes to osteoarthrosis but the precise relationship cannot be established. It will cause stiffness and pain. The presence of a posterior tibial fragment, in the so called trimalleolar fracture, implies considerable violence and adversely affects prognosis. Even when the fragment is small and extra-articular, osteoarthrosis occurs in 17% of patients. When the fragment is large and involves the articular surface, the incidence of osteoarthrosis increases to 30% even when reduction is exact, and to 45% if malunion is present.

Osteoarthrosis of the ankle is found in 20–40% of patients after ankle fractures (Wilson and Skilbred, 1966). It can develop after union in anatomical position, although rarely (less than 10%). It becomes increasingly common as the extent of residual displacement increases, but the relationship is not mathematical (Pettrone *et al.,* 1983). Osteoarthrosis becomes apparent on X-ray within 18 months of union and does not appear after this time.

There is an association between the severity of osteoarthrosis and the clinical result. If narrowing of the joint space is used as the criterion of severity, it has been shown that when the joint space has been reduced by 50% over half the patients have a poor clinical result. When the joint space is almost obliterated a poor clinical result is inevitable.

Age of the patient

The results of displaced fractures are worse after the age of 50, particularly in postmenopausal women (Beauchamp, Clay and Thexton, 1983).

Prognosis

1. A provisional prognosis can be given at the onset of treatment, based on the severity of the injury and the age of the patient. Some 30% of all patients will experience discomfort after 5 years.
2. An interim prognosis can be given at the end of treatment based on the quality of the reduction.
3. A definitive prognosis can be given 18 months later based on the presence of osteoarthrosis as shown by decrease in joint space. The incidence of arthrosis will not increase thereafter (Lindsjo, 1981).

Fractures of the lower articular surface of the tibia

These injuries have recently been described as plafond or pylon fractures. A plafond is an archaic French word meaning a ceiling, and is now an artistic term used to describe a painting on a ceiling. In archaeological terms a pylon is the monumental gateway to an Egyptian temple formed by truncated pyramids connected by a lower architectural member containing the gate (*Shorter Oxford English Dictionary*, 1978). One can object, on aesthetic grounds, against the use of these words to describe articular fractures of the lower tibia, but probably in vain and they are here to stay.

The prognosis of these fractures depends on the accuracy of their reduction. Malunion, including particularly widening of the ankle mortice, predisposes to osteoarthrosis (Ovadia and Beals, 1986).

Fractures of the ankle in children

Fractures involving epiphyses and growth plate have been classified by Salter and Harris (1963) This classification, as applied to fractures around the ankle in children, has been modified by

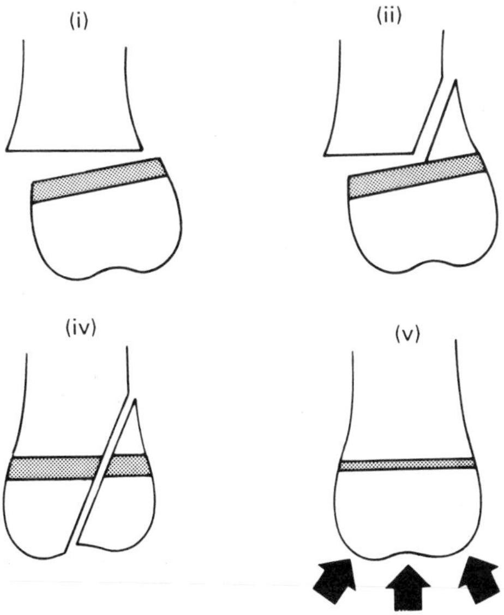

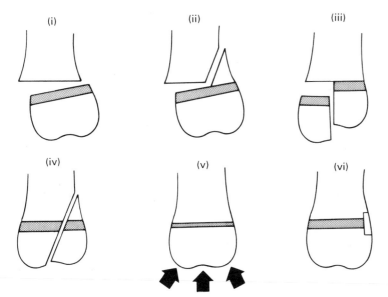

Figure 51.1 Salter/Harris classification of epiphyseal injuries

Chadwick and Bentley (1987) to allow a firm prognosis soon after injury.

The Salter/Harris classification describes six types of injury (see Figure 51.1). Damage to the growth plate can result in retardation of growth causing either angular deformity from unequal growth or true shortening. Malunion involving the articular surface can lead to osteoarthrosis in later life.

Chadwick and Bentley (1987) suggested four groups of ankle fractures in children.

Table 51.1 Classification of ankle fractures in children

Chadwick/Bentley	*Salter/Harris*	*Prognosis*
I	I or II	No retardation of growth
II (Displaced laterally)	III or IV	No retardation
III (Displaced medially)	III or IV	Retardation
IV Crush injuries	V	Retardation

References

Beauchamp, C. G., Clay, N. R. and Thexton, P. W. (1983) Displaced ankle fractures in patients over 50 years of age. *Journal of Bone and Joint Surgery,* **65B**, 329–332

Chadwick, C. J. and Bentley, G. (1987) The classification and prognosis of epiphyseal injuries. *Injury,* **18**, 157–168

Lindsjo, J. (1981) Operative treatment of ankle fractures. *Acta Orthopaedica Scandinavia,* **52**, 189

Mendelsohn, H. A. (1965) Non-union of malleolar fractures of the ankle. *Clinical Orthopaedics,* **42**, 103–118

Ovadia, D. N. and Beals, R. K. (1986) Fractures of the tibial plafond. *Journal of Bone and Joint Surgery,* **68A**, 543–551

Pettrone, F. A., Gail, M., Pee, D., Fitzpatrick, T. and Van Herbe, L. B. (1983) Quantitative criteria for prediction of the results of displaced ankle fractures. *Journal of Bone and Joint Surgery,* **65A**, 667–677

Phillips, W. A., Schwartz, H. S., Keller, C. S. *et al.* (1985) A prospective randomised study of the management of severe ankle fractures. *Journal of Bone and Joint Surgery,* **67A**, 67–78

Salter, R. B. and Harris, W. (1963) Injuries involving the epiphyseal plate. *Journal of Bone and Joint Surgery,* **45A**, 587–622

Sarkisian, J. S. and Cody, S. W. (1976) Closed treatment of ankle fractures. *Journal of Trauma,* **16**, 323–326

Wilson, F. C. and Skilbred, L. A. (1966) Long term results in treatment of displaced bi-malleolar fractures. *Journal of Bone and Joint Surgery,* **48A**, 1065–1078

Table 51.2

Injury	Fractures of the medial malleolus
Structural impairment	Non-union. 1% (ORIF) 20% (Conservative)
Subjective impairment	Local discomfort
Disability and handicap	Minimal
Comments	

Table 51.3

Injury	Bimalleolar fractures of the ankle
Structural impairment	Non-union of medial malleolus Malunion Osteoarthrosis of ankle joint – less than 10% if reduction is anatomical
Subjective impairment	Pain Stiffness – limp Swelling Deformity
Disability and handicap	Limited ability to walk, climb stairs, drive vehicles
Comments	Osteoarthrosis apparent by 18 months

Table 51.4

Injury	Trimalleolar fractures of the ankle
Structural impairment	Malunion Osteoarthrosis – 17% with small, extra-articular fragment 20% with reduced large fragment 45% with malunion
Subjective impairment	Pain Stiffness Swelling Deformity
Disability and handicap	Disability can be severe and may lead to arthrodesis of the ankle joint
Comments	Severe handicap in weight-bearing occupations and sport Choice of footwear limited Provisional prognosis can be given when first seen; 30% possibility of residual symptoms

Table 51.5

Injury	Fractures of the lower articular surface of the tibia
Structural impairment	Malunion – will result in symptomatic osteoarthrosis if mortice widening is more than 2 mm or if fragments are laterally displaced by more than 5 mm Osteoarthrosis
Subjective impairment	Pain Stiffness due to osteoarthrosis in 20% (5% severe enough to warrant arthrodesis) Swelling *But* normal movement in less than 70%
Disability and handicap	84% likely to return to pre-accident occupation 54% likely to return to sport
Comments	Result depends on accuracy of reduction AO fixation can result in 90% with no malunion

Table 51.6

Injury	Fractures of the ankle in children
Structural impairment	*Growth retardation* Chadwick/Bentley I No impairment II No impairment III Growth retardation. Varus deformity IV Growth retardation. Shortening less than 2 cm Malunion – late osteoarthrosis if articular step greater than 2 mm
Subjective impairment	Varus deformity causing pain and limp
Disability and handicap	Shortening not a cause of disability Osteoarthrosis in an adult may cause pain and stiffness
Comments	In Group III and IV (above) observation should continue for 2 years before a definitive prognosis is given

52
Rupture of the lateral ligament of the ankle

Reviews suggest that the long-term results of effective conservative treatment of this injury are as good as those of immediate operative repair (Evans, Hardcastle and Frenyo, 1984). If the instability is untreated, the incidence of late osteoarthrosis is 100%, but symptoms may not arise for 10 years (Harrington, 1979). The long-term results of tenodesis for chronic instability are not as good as those achieved by adequate primary treatment of the injury (Van der Rijt and Evans, 1984).

References

Evans, G. A., Hardcastle, P. and Frenyo, A. D. (1984) Acute rupture of the lateral ligament of the ankle. *Journal of Bone and Joint Surgery,* **66B**, 209–212

Harrington, K. D. (1979) Degenerative arthritis of the ankle secondary to long-standing lateral ligament instability. *Journal of Bone and Joint Surgery,* **61A**, 354–361

Van der Rijt, A. J. and Evans, G. A. (1984) The long-term results of Watson-Jones tenodesis. *Journal of Bone and Joint Surgery,* **66B**, 371–375

Table 52.1

Injury	Rupture of lateral ligament of the ankle
Structural impairment	Slack lateral ligament of the ankle Tilting of the talus Osteoarthrosis of ankle – 100% in untreated cases
Subjective impairment	Pain Swelling Stiffness Difficulty in walking over uneven ground 'Giving way'
Disability and handicap	No significant long-term disability in spite of persisting symptoms All reviewed patients returned to pre-accident employment after Watson-Jones tenodesis
Comments	Energetic primary treatment, conservative or operative, gives better long-term results than tenodesis for chronic instability

53

Rupture of the Achilles tendon

This is an injury of the middle aged, often missed as an early diagnosis. Untreated, the patient is left with a flat-footed limp. Successful operative treatment ensures a return to functional normality but wasting of the calf muscles is permanent. Conservative treatment avoids the complications of wound infection and dehiscence but recurrence of rupture occurs in 10% of injuries so treated (Hooker, 1963; Lea and Smith, 1972).

References

Hooker, C. H. (1963) Rupture of the tendo-calcaneus. *Journal of Bone and Joint Surgery,* **45B**, 360–363

Lea, R. B. and Smith, L. (1972) Non-surgical treatment of tendo Achilles rupture. *Journal of Bone and Joint Surgery,* **54A**, 1398–1403

54

Fractures and fracture dislocations of the talus

The talus is injured by forces transmitted through the sole of the foot, often accompanied by a twisting component which can displace the talus from the ankle mortice or the other bones of the foot from the talus. If the injuries are graded in severity, as by Kenright and Taylor (1970), the incidence of residual disability ranges from 0 to 75%. More precise classification allows clear prognosis for specific types of injury, as talar fractures have been the subject of many detailed reviews. The following groups will be considered:

1. Fractures of the peripheral processes, including the lateral process.
2. Fractures of the neck of the talus.
3. Fractures of the body of the talus.
4. Osteochondral fractures of the talus.
5. Dislocation of the talus.
6. Subtalar dislocation.

Earlier reviews, including Coltart's classic 'Aviators' astragalus' (1952) which reviewed 228 cases from the RAF, gave an overall complication rate of 70–80%.

Fractures of the lateral process

These seemingly minor fractures can be a potent source of residual disability if they are not recognized and energetically treated. Hawkins (1965) reviewed 13 cases and found six had malunion or non-union, causing pain, stiffness and swelling. The diagnosis had been missed on first presentation in six of the patients he reviewed. Mukherjee, Pringle and Baxter (1974) also described 13 cases and again found six with residual symptoms, four of them having severe pain.

Fractures of the neck of the talus

Hawkins' (1970) classification of these fractures into three types has become accepted: Hawkins Type I is undisplaced fracture; Hawkins Type II is displaced fracture with subtalar subluxation; Hawkins Type III is displaced fracture with dislocation of the body of the talus. This particular injury is fraught with complications and associated with a high incidence of residual impairment. The most common impairment is avascular necrosis of the body of the talus, occurring in up to 80% of Type III fractures. Hawkins (1970) described the following sign which is useful in forecasting this. A subchondral radiolucent line in the dome of the talus, visible at 6–8 weeks after injury, is reliable evidence that the blood supply to the body is intact. Radiographic evidence of bone death, increased bone density, may not be apparent for 3 months. Canale and Kelly (1978) found this sign not to be totally reliable, with a 5% incidence of false reading. Other complications include malunion, non-union and late osteoarthrosis.

Fractures of the body of the talus

These are less common, comprising 22 out of Coltart's 228 cases. Malunion, avascular necrosis and late osteoarthrosis can occur (Coltart, 1952; Kenwright and Taylor, 1970).

Osteochondral fractures of the talus

If these fractures resulted in the formation of a loose body, residual symptoms including a painful limp and later osteoarthrosis appeared in 34 of 68 cases reviewed by Pettine and Morrey (1987).

Dislocation of the talus

This gross injury, usually compound, leaves severe residual disability. The reduced talus does not survive in half the patients and one of the nine cases described by Detenbeck and Kelly (1969) came to below-knee amputation.

Subtalar dislocation

Dislocation of the tarsus from the talus is a gross injury but the results are surprisingly good unless the dislocation is compound (Monson and Ryan, 1981; DeLee and Curtis, 1982) with a zero rate of avascular necrosis. Residual symptoms of pain and stiffness due to a 50% rate of osteoarthrosis stabilize within 2 years and give rise to significant disability in a minority.

References

Canale, S. T. and Kelly, F. B. (1978) Fractures of the neck of the talus. *Journal of Bone and Joint Surgery,* **60A**, 143–156

Coltart, D. (1952) Aviators' astragalus. *Journal of Bone and Joint Surgery,* **34B**, 542–566

DeLee, J. C. and Curtis, R. (1982) Subtalar dislocation of the foot. *Journal of Bone and Joint Surgery,* **64A**, 433–437

Detenbeck, L. C. and Kelly, P. J. (1969) Total dislocation of the talus. *Journal of Bone and Joint Surgery,* **51A**, 283–288

Hawkins, L. G. (1965) Fractures of lateral process of the talus. *Journal of Bone and Joint Surgery,* **47A**, 1170–1175

Hawkins, L. G. (1970) Fractures of the neck of the talus. *Journal of Bone and Joint Surgery,* **52A**, 991–1002

Kenwright, J. and Taylor, R. G. (1970) Major injuries of the talus. *Journal of Bone and Joint Surgery,* **52B**, 36–48

Monson, S. T. and Ryan, J. R. (1981) Subtalar dislocation. *Journal of Bone and Joint Surgery,* **63A**, 1156–1158

Mukherjee, S. K., Pringle, R. M. and Baxter, A. D. (1974) Fracture of lateral process of talus. *Journal of Bone and Joint Surgery,* **56B**, 263–273

Pettine, K. A. and Morrey, B. F. (1987) Osteochondral fractures of the talus. *Journal of Bone and Joint Surgery,* **69B**, 89–92

Table 54.1

Injury	Fractures of the lateral and posterior processes of the talus
Structural impairment	Malunion (including overgrowth) Non-union } 45% } Pain Stiffness Swelling } 25% mild 25% severe enough to warrant treatment
Subjective impairment	Painful limp Over half have no symptoms 3 months after injury
Disability and handicap	Limitation on standing, walking, running, climbing
Comments	Definitive prognosis should be deferred until 18 months after injury, as disability will either resolve or become established by then

Table 54.2

Injury	Fractures of the neck of the talus – undisplaced (Hawkins Type I)
Structural impairment	Malunion 0% Non-union 0% Avascular necrosis 0% (Hawkins) 13% (Canale and Kelly) 4% overall Osteoarthrosis (ankle or subtalar) 15–25%
Subjective impairment	Painful limp
Disability and handicap	Handicapped for standing, walking, running, climbing } 10% Good clinical result in 90%
Comments	

Table 54.3

Injury	Fractures of the neck of the talus – displaced (Hawkins Type II)
Structural impairment	Malunion 15 of 53 and 18 of 71 (26%) Non-union 0–7% (including delayed union) Avascular necrosis 42–50% Osteoarthrosis of ankle 36% Subtalar osteoarthrosis 66%
Subjective impairment	Painful limp in over 60% of cases
Disability and handicap	Handicapped in standing, walking, running, climbing } over 60%
Comments	Prolonged non-weight bearing can reduce residual disability in avascular necross to 11% (Canale and Kelly) Accurate reduction and internal fixation eliminates malunion and reduces disability from osteoarthrosis

Table 54.4

Injury	Fractures of neck of talus – displaced with dislocation of body (Hawkins Type III)
Structural impairment	Malunion 12% Non-union 5% Avascular necrosis 90% Osteoarthrosis of ankle 70% Subtalar osteoarthrosis 65%
Subjective impairment	Severe pain and limp in 75%
Disability and handicap	Patient unlikely to return to heavy physical work
Comments	Subtalar osteoarthrosis is the impairment most productive of disability Avascular necrosis alone does not result in disability in nearly 30% of those affected

Table 54.5

Injury	Fractures of the body of the talus
Structural impairment	Malunion 100% Avascular necrosis 30% Osteoarthrosis of ankle } Over 60% Subtalar osteoarthrosis }
Subjective impairment	Painful limp, severe in 75%
Disability and handicap	
Comments	

Table 54.6

Injury	Osteochondral fractures of talus
Structural impairment	Loose body 39% (detached fragment)
Subjective impairment	Painful limp and swelling 76% Symptoms incapacitating in 25%
Disability and handicap	
Comments	Symptoms become stable 1 year after treatment

Table 54.7

Injury	Subtalar dislocation
Structural impairment	Avascular necrosis – <5% Osteoarthrosis – 40% (Peritalar)
Subjective impairment	Pain, stiffness and limp in 45%
Disability and handicap	Handicapped in climbing and walking over rough ground in over 50%
Comments	The results in the short term are good, but fall off with time Prognosis should be guarded for 2 years

Table 54.8

Injury	Total dislocation of talus
Structural impairment	Avascular necrosis Infection Peritalar osteoarthrosis
Subjective impairment	Severe permanent disability almost certain Nearly all come to talectomy or talocalcaneal fusion At best the foot will be stiff There is a 10% risk of below-knee amputation
Disability and handicap	Permanently handicapped for heavy physical work
Comments	The injury is often compound when first seen or becomes so from pressure necrosis of skin Treatment is salvage

55

Fractures of the calcaneum

The prognosis of fractures of the calcaneum depends on the extent of damage sustained by the subtalar joint, and is assisted by a classification of degrees of severity. The following groups have been used: Group I, fractures of the body of the calcaneus; Group II, comminuted fractures without subtalar depression; Group III, depression of the subtalar joint (Nade and Monaghan, 1972).

The deformity can be measured on the lateral radiograph by drawing the tuber–joint angle (Bohler, 1931).

Fractures not involving the subtalar joint result in a satisfactory outcome in nearly all patients. Over 90% return to work within 3 months and fewer than 10% have any residual symptoms (Essex-Lopresti, 1952; Nade and Monaghan, 1972).

Reported results in patients with articular fractures vary. Much argument has arisen over the merits of various methods of treatment, ranging from the frankly nihilistic approaches of accepting the deformity and either encouraging early movement or arthrodesing the damaged joint as a primary treatment, to open reduction and internal fixation based on detailed analysis of the displaced fragments.

Pozo, Kirwan and Jackson (1984) reviewed 21 patients with depressed fractures treated by active mobilization. They found that after a minimum follow up of 8 years, 76% had minor residual symptoms. They also found that a quarter of their patients continued to improve for up to 6 years after injury.

Persistent pain and stiffness, of varying severity, is reported in a majority of patients with depressed fractures. These symptoms arise from osteoarthrosis of the subtalar joint or adhesions of the peroneal tendons. Other impairments affecting the result are loss of heel height, broadening of the heel and swelling. The high incidence of such impairment emerges in all reports, but what also emerges is that the majority of patients return to heavy work (Roberts, 1950; Barnard and Odegaard, 1970; Nade and

Monaghan, 1972). Most reports show little improvement occurring after 2 years.

Subtalar stiffness, of course, imposes a peculiar handicap on those whose occupation takes them across uneven ground or on to scaffolding and ladders. A change of occupation may be necessary (in 14% of Nade and Monaghan's patients). Age has an adverse effect. Essex-Lopresti (1952) found marked deterioration in patients over middle age.

References

Barnard, L. and Odegaard, J. K. (1970) Fractures of calcaneum. *Journal of Bone and Joint Surgery,* **52A**, 1689

Bohler, L. (1931) Pathology and treatment of fractures of the os calcis. *Journal of Bone and Joint Surgery,* **13**, 75–89

Essex-Lopresti, P. (1952) The mechanism, reduction technique and results in fractures of the os calcis. *British Journal of Surgery,* **39**, 395–419

Nade, S. and Monaghan, P. R. W. (1972) Fractures of the calcaneus. *Journal of Bone and Joint Surgery,* **54B**, 177

Noble, J. and McQuillan, W. M. (1979) Early posterior fusion in the treatment of fractures of the os calcis. *Journal of Bone and Joint Surgery,* **61B**, 90

Pozo, J. L., Kirwan, E. O. and Jackson, A. M. (1984) Long term results of conservative management of severely displaced fractures of the calcaneus. *Journal of Bone and Joint Surgery,* **66B**, 386–390

Roberts, N. (1950) Fractures of the calcaneus. *Journal of Bone and Joint Surgery,* **50B**, 884

Table 55.1

Injury	Grade I extra-articular and Grade II undisplaced fractures of the calcaneum
Structural impairment	Osteoarthrosis of subtalar joint occurs in up to 40% of Grade II fractures
Subjective impairment	Pain Stiffness
Disability and handicap	Impaired ability to walk over uneven surfaces Overall results of extra-articular fractures over 90% good Overall results of undisplaced fractures affecting the subtalar joint 70–75% good
Comments	

Table 55.2

Injury	Grade III depressed fractures involving the subtalar joint
Structural impairment	Fibrous ankylosis and osteoarthrosis of subtalar joint Deformity of heel including loss of height, broadening, valgus deformity and atrophy of heel pad
Subjective impairment	Pain, Stiffness, Swelling } – 65–90%
Disability and handicap	Restricted ability to walk over rough ground or sloping surfaces Results adversely affected by age
Comments	Subtalar stiffness alone need not constitute a handicap. Noble and McQuillan (1979) reported 94% good or excellen results in 47 patients treated by primary subtalar fusion through a posterior approach

56

Midtarsal injuries

Main and Jowett (1975) describe 18 varieties of midtarsal injury ranging from simple sprains to complex fracture dislocations. Included are displaced fractures of the navicular which merit separate consideration from the point of view of prognosis. The other injuries include soft tissue sprains and undisplaced fractures which do well with simple conservative measures, leaving no residual disability. Dislocations and fracture dislocations of the midtarsal joints often require open reduction and the overall results show a 50% incidence of residual disability in the form of pain and stiffness (Wilson, 1982).

References

Main, B. J. and Jowett, T. (1975) Injuries of the midtarsal joint. *Journal of Bone and Joint Surgery,* **57B**, 89–97

Wilson, D. W. (1982) Fractures of the foot. In *The Foot and its Disorders*, 2nd edn (ed. L. Klenerman), Blackwell Scientific Publications, Oxford, pp. 272–283

Displaced fractures of the navicular

These uncommon fractures are often missed. Recent reports suggest that results can be improved by open reduction and internal fixation of displaced fragments (Sangeorzan *et al.*, 1989).

The results of closed treatment are poor, with a high incidence of malunion and avascular necrosis leading to residual pain and stiffness (Eichenholtz and Levine, 1964; Eftekhar, Lyddon and Stevens, 1969).

References

Eichenholtz, S. N. and Levine, D. B. (1964) Fractures of the tarsal navicular. *Clinical Orthopaedics,* **34**, 142–157

Eftekhar, N. M., Lyddon, D. W. and Stevens, J. (1969) Unusual fracture-dislocations of the tarsal navicular. *Journal of Bone and Joint Surgery,* **51A**, 577–581

Sangeorzan, B. J., Benirschke, S. K., Mosca, V., Mayo, K. A. and Hansen, S. T. (1989) Displaced intra-articular fractures of the tarsal navicular. *Journal of Bone and Joint Surgery,* **71A**, 1504–1510

Table 56.1

Injury	Displaced fractures of the navicular
Structural impairment	Malunion 33% Avascular necrosis 30% Osteoarthrosis 33%
Subjective impairment	Overall results are poor with over 30% of patients complaining of residual pain and stiffness (restricted pronation and supination) Less than 20% are completely symptom free at 1 year
Disability and handicap	Handicapped in standing walking running working on rough ground
Comments	These are uncommon injuries, with varying degrees of severity. The less severe fractures are often missed and residual disability may follow delay in treatment. Good results are established by 1 year, so prognosis need not be delayed further.

57

Fracture and fracture dislocations of the tarsometatarsal joints

The risk of damage to the dorsalis pedis artery led Gissane to call Lisfranc's fracture dislocation 'a dangerous type of fracture' (Gissane, 1951), but arterial damage is a rare complication of this injury being found in but two patients out of 119 in a multicentre review (Hardcastle *et al.*, 1982). The incidence of post-traumatic osteoarthrosis has been reported as 23% (Jeffreys, 1963) to 100% (Wilson, 1972; Hardcastle *et al.*, 1982). All authors agree that there is no correlation between the radiographic appearances of osteoarthrosis and the patient's symptoms, but opinions differ as to the relevance of anatomical reduction to the functional result. Some believe that a good result depends on accurate reduction (Wilson, 1972; Le Gay and Amirault, 1989), while others feel that it makes little difference (Jeffreys, 1963; Brunet and Wiley, 1987).

Most patients have residual symptoms of pain and stiffness. The clinical picture can take 1–5 years to stabilize but 70% of all patients lead a normal life with minimal symptoms (Brunet and Wiley, 1987). A residual deformity of the foot can make the fitting of footwear difficult, and this forced a change of occupation in three out of Wilson's 22 patients, and in six of the 33 reviewed by Brunet and Wiley.

References

Brunet, J. A. and Wiley, J. J. (1987) Late results of tarsometatarsal joint injuries. *Journal of Bone and Joint Surgery*, **69B**, 437–440

Gissane, W. (1951) A dangerous type of fracture of the foot. *Journal of Bone and Joint Surgery*, **33B**, 535–538

Hardcastle, P. H., Reschauer, R., Kulsha-Linsberg, E. and Schoffman, W. (1982) Injuries to the tarsometatarsal joint. *Journal of Bone and Joint Surgery*, **64B**, 349–356

Jeffreys, T. E. (1963) Lisfranc's fracture-dislocation. *Journal of Bone and Joint Surgery*, **45B**, 546–551

Le Gay, D. A. and Amirault, J. D. (1989) Tarsometatarsal joint injuries. *Orthopaedic Transactions*, **13**(3), 654–655

Wilson, D. W. (1972) Injuries of the tarsometatarsal joints. *Journal of Bone and Joint Surgery*, **54B**, 677–686

Table 57.1

Injury	Tarsometatarsal fracture dislocations
Structural impairment	Malunion Osteoarthrosis 23–100%
Subjective impairment	Pain Stiffness up to 95% Deformity. May be so severe as to prevent footwear fitting No patients totally symptom free
Disability and handicap	Over 75% of patients are able to return to their pre-accident occupation
Comments	Overall functional results – good, 67%; fair, 23.5%; poor, 8.8% (Hardcastle) There is disagreement as to the influence of accurate reduction on prognosis, but unreduced injuries result in severe disability Clinical result may take 1–5 years to stabilize

58

Fractures of the fifth metatarsal

Robert Jones commented on the incidence of non-union of fractures of the base of the fifth metatarsal, having suffered the injury himself (Jones, 1902). More recently it has become recognized as an injury with disabling results in athletes (Dameron, 1975; Kavanaugh, Brower and Mann, 1978). Avulsion fractures of the tuberosity unite readily with no residual problems unless they are associated with injuries of the ankle (Pearson, 1961).

References

Dameron, T. B. (1975) Fracture and anatomical variations of the proximal portion of the fifth metatarsal. *Journal of Bone and Joint Surgery,* **57A**, 788–792

Kavanaugh, J. H., Brower, T. D. and Mann, R. V. (1978) The Jones fracture revisited. *Journal of Bone and Joint Surgery,* **60A**, 776–782

Jones, R. (1902) Fracture of the base of the fifth metatarsal by indirect violence. *Annals of Surgery,* **35**, 697–700

Pearson, J. R. (1961) Combined fracture of the base of the fifth metatarsal and the lateral malleolus. *Journal of Bone and Joint Surgery,* **43A**, 513–516

Table 58.1

Injury	Fractures of the fifth metatarsal
Structural impairment	Delayed union 66% (Kavanaugh) 25% (Torg) Non-union 20% (Torg)
Subjective impairment	Pain
Disability and handicap	Limitation of sporting activities
Comments	The Jones fracture is often not recognized as such, and is not seen until delayed or non-union are radiologically apparent. The fracture must then be grafted

59
Injuries of the forefoot

Fractures of the forefoot are common industrial injuries resulting from a heavy weight being dropped on the foot. The wearing of industrial boots with steel toe caps has reduced the frequency of phalangeal fractures, but they do not protect the metatarsus. In some European countries the metal extends more proximal (R. Schubert, personal communication) and the old wooden clog or sabot provides even more protection. Metatarsal and phalangeal fractures heal readily, although painless fibrous union often occurs in the toes. Residual pain after forefoot fractures may persist for 12–18 months. Metatarsalgia can follow malunited fractures of the necks of metatarsals (Watson-Jones, 1956).

Prognosis depends more on the degree of soft tissue damage, which may be extensive with necrosis and loss of skin, peri-articular scarring and adhesion of tendons.

References

Watson-Jones, R. (1956) *Fractures and Joint Injuries,* 4th edn, E. & S. Livingstone, Edinburgh, pp. 905

Part 4

Peripheral nerve injuries

60

Injuries of peripheral nerves

There are four recognized forms of peripheral nerve lesions.

1. *Neurapraxia*. Conduction along the nerve is interrupted but there is no loss of structural continuity. The neurological defect is always incomplete and complete recovery is to be expected within weeks. Nerve lesions associated with closed fractures are usually of this type. A confident prognosis of recovery can be made; and management is expectant.
2. *Axonotmesis*. The nerve sheath is intact but there is axonal disruption within the sheath. The injury is produced by traction.
3. *Neurotmesis*. The nerve is completely divided. The injury occurs in open wounds. Partial recovery of function follows operative apposition and repair (Seddon, 1942).
4. A fourth variety of injury has recently been described, where the myelin of the nerve sheath is dispersed by external pressure but the axon remains intact. Release of the pressure is followed by rapid recovery. It has been called *axonamonosis* (Birch and Strange, 1990).

References

Birch, R. and Strange, F. G. St. C. (1990) A new type of peripheral nerve lesion. *Journal of Bone and Joint Surgery, 72B*, 312–313

Seddon, H. J. (1942) A classification of nerve injuries. *British Medical Journal,* **ii**, 237–239

Brachial plexus lesions

Brachial plexus lesions are uncommon and should be managed by surgeons with particular interest and experience in their problems.

The injury occurs in young male victims of high-velocity road accidents and early definitive prognosis is important in planning rehabilitation. It has been shown that prognosis can be settled as early as 8 weeks after injury (Ransford and Hughes, 1977). The prognosis is based on the following evidence:

1. A high-velocity injury implies extensive root damage.
2. Severe persistent pain implies a bad prognosis, but being subjective is in itself unreliable.
3. A Horners syndrome is usually a bad sign.
4. The presence of normal axon reflexes, as shown by histamine testing, in an area of skin supplied by a nerve of the brachial plexus implies that the lesion of that nerve is proximal to the posterior root ganglion, and has probably been avulsed from the cord rendering recovery impossible. The test must be delayed for 3 weeks after injury to allow axonal degeneration to occur (Bonney, 1959).
5. Multiple traumatic meningoceles on cervical myelography imply root avulsion and indicate a bad prognosis. Single meningoceles must be interpreted with caution (Yeoman, 1968).

An interesting observation in the 10-year follow up of 20 cases of complete brachial plexus lesions by Ransford and Hughes was that the development of cervical spondylosis was not accelerated in these patients.

The place of Magnetic Resonance Injury in prognosis is unknown as yet.

The prognosis for those found to have complete lesions is poor. Recent attempts at surgical reconstruction have resulted in some improvement in shoulder function but none in small muscle function or useful sensation in the hand (Barton, 1987). Sedel (1982) reported results from surgical repair that were distinctly better than no treatment at all. Of his operated patients, 14% were able to do manual work, and only 19% finished with a completely useless arm. Nearly 50% of his conservatively treated patients were left with an arm that was useless.

References

Barton, N. J. (1987) Brachial plexus lesions. In *Neuromuscular Problems in Orthopaedics* (ed. C. S. B. Galasko), Blackwells Scientific Publishers, pp. 218–223

Bonney, G. (1959) Prognosis in traction lesions of the brachial plexus. *Journal of Bone and Joint Surgery,* **41B**, 4–35

Ransford, A. O. and Hughes, S. P. F. (1977) Complete brachial plexus lesions. *Journal of Bone and Joint Surgery,* **59B**, 417–420

Sedel, L. (1982) The results of surgical repair of brachial plexus injuries. *Journal of Bone and Joint Surgery,* **64B**, 54–66

Yeoman, P. M. (1968) Cervical myelography in traction injuries of the brachial plexus. *Journal of Bone and Joint Surgery,* **50B**, 253–260

Table 60.1

Injury	Complete lesions of brachial plexus	
Structural impairment **Subjective impairment**	Complete motor paralysis and sensory loss of upper limb Pain	
Disability and handicap	*Results graded by Sedel* (modified by Barton) (usefulness of limb function)	%
	Grade 1, manual work with normal strength	0
	Grade 2, able to help in everyday activities	18
	Grade 3, functions only as hook or paperweight	35
	Grade 4, useless but some movement	4
	Grade 5, no movement and no use	43
Comments	Prognosis firm at 8 weeks High-velocity injury Persistent pain Horners syndrome Axon reflexes Multiple meningoceles } if all positive, no recovery	

Peripheral nerve injuries in the upper limb

Circumflex nerve (axillary nerve)

The nerve is injured during anterior dislocation of the shoulder joint. The reported incidence varies from 5.5% (Rowe, 1956) to 18% (Hawkins *et al.*, 1986). Between 15 and 30% of these do not recover but the prognosis deteriorates with age; recovery is to be expected in patients under 50 years of age (Pasila *et al.*, 1980). Recovery can occur up to 1 year after injury.

References

Hawkins, R. J., Bell, R. H., Hawkins, R. H. and Koppert, G. J. (1986) Anterior dislocation of the shoulder in the older patient. *Clinical Orthopaedics,* **206**, 192–195

Pasila, M., Kiviluoto, O., Jaroma, H. and Sundholm, A. (1980) Recovery from primary shoulder dislocation and its complications. *Acta Orthopaedica Scandinavia,* **51**, 257–262

Rowe, C. R. (1956) Prognosis in dislocations of the shoulder. *Journal of Bone and Joint Surgery,* **38A**, 957–977

Radial nerve

Closed injury to the radial nerve is associated with fractures of the shaft of the humerus in up to 18% of cases (Mast *et al.*, 1975). The reported rate of recovery varies from 50% (Sim, Kelly and Henderson, 1971) to 100% (Pollock *et al.*, 1981). The lesion is usually in continuity and it is advisable to allow 8–10 weeks for recovery to occur before exploration. Sim and his colleagues, however, advocated exploration within 3 weeks.

Posterior interosseous nerve lesions can follow injury to the head of the radius, particularly the Monteggia fracture dislocation. Recovery is to be expected.

References

Mast, J. W., Spiegel, P. G., Harvey, J. P. and Harrison, C. (1975) Fractures of the humeral shaft. *Clinical Orthopaedics,* **112**, 254–262

Pollock, F. H., Drake, D., Bovill, E. G., Day, L. and Trafton, P. G. (1981) Treatment of radial neuropathy associated with fractures of the humerus. *Journal of Bone and Joint Surgery,* **63A**, 239–243

Sim, F. H., Kelly, P. J. and Henderson, E. D. (1971) Radial nerve palsy complicating fractures of the humeral shaft. *Journal of Bone and Joint Surgery,* **53A**, 1023

Median nerve

The median nerve can be injured in association with fractures from the humerus down, in association with Volkmann's ischaemic contracture, and in open wounds of the forearm or wrist. It is the sensory nerve of the hand and its loss is disabling. The most common fracture causing the lesion is the Colles' fracture, but it is also seen after supracondylar fractures in children. After Colles' fracture it can occur acutely or it can present later as a carpal tunnel syndrome (Stewart, Innes and Burke, 1985). When median injury complicates supracondylar fracture, the lesion is usually in continuity, although it may require release by open reduction of the fracture. The median nerve may be damaged by ischaemia and compressed by fibrosis of the muscle infarct in Volkmann's contracture.

Open division of the median nerve in the forearm or at the wrist deprives most of the hand of sensation and paralyses the small muscles of the thumb. This loss is grievious. In the AMA *Guides to Evaluation*, total median loss is graded as 73% impairment of the upper limb, and 44% impairment of the whole arm if the dominant limb is affected.

Repair of any peripheral nerve never results in 100% return of function. Results are better in the younger patient. Full recovery may take up to 18 months to be complete. There will be some degree of permanent impairment of sensation, and this is particularly disabling in median nerve injuries. The most optimistic expectation will be about 70% of normal (Mackenzie and Woods, 1961). Using the AMA criteria this leaves 55% impairment of upper limb function. Function continues to improve for up to 4 years after repair (Nicholson and Seddon, 1957).

These are crude figures, and prognosis for function must take into account the patient's age, his or her occupation and leisure activities and whether the dominant hand is affected. Assessment of the end result is difficult and varies between examiners (Marsh and Barton, 1987).

References

American Medical Association (1977) *Guides to the Evaluation of Permanent Impairment*, pp. 49–59

Mackenzie, I. G. and Woods, C. G. (1961) Causes of failure after repair of the median nerve. *Journal of Bone and Joint Surgery,* **43B**, 465–473

Marsh, D. and Barton, N. J. (1987) Does the operating microscope improve the results of peripheral nerve suture? *Journal of Bone and Joint Surgery,* **69B**, 625–630

Nicholson, O. R. and Seddon, H. J. (1957) Nerve repair in civil practice. *British Medical Journal,* **ii**, 1065–1071
Stewart, H. D., Innes, A. R. and Burke, F. D. (1985) The hand complications of Colles' fracture. *Journal of Hand Surgery,* **10B**, 103–106

Ulnar nerve

The ulnar nerve may be injured by compression, at the elbow or in the hand. It can be injured in fractures around the elbow, forearm or wrist. These nerve injuries are almost invariably in continuity, with excellent prospects of spontaneous recovery.

Division of the ulnar nerve at the wrist causes paralysis of the small muscles of the hand and loss of sensation in the little finger and the adjacent surface of the ring finger. Total ulnar paralysis is not as catastrophic as the median lesion because the sensory defect is not as important. The AMA Guide rates it as causing 33% impairment of the upper limb, 20% of the whole man, if the dominant limb is affected. It must be remembered, however, that the ulnar nerve is 'the nerve of the power grip' (Bowden and Napier, 1961) and an ulnar nerve lesion may constitute more of a disability in an unskilled manual labourer than in a craftsman.

Reference

Bowden, R. E. M. and Napier, J. R. (1961) The assessment of hand function after peripheral nerve injuries. *Journal of Bone and Joint Surgery,* **43B**, 481–492

Digital nerves

Digital nerves are purely sensory nerves and good results after suture can be expected. Recovery is always imperfect but this is of functional significance only if the tip of the thumb and the tip of the index finger are numb (Bowden and Napier, 1961). Neuromata formation and cold intolerance are common, as they are after any peripheral nerve lesion. The AMA assessment varies from 8% impairment of the upper limb, if the tip of the thumb is anaesthetic, to 2%, if sensation is lost over the tip of the little finger.

References

Bowden, R. E. M. and Napier, J. R. (1961) The assessment of hand function after peripheral nerve injuries. *Journal of Bone and Joint Surgery,* **43B**, 481–492

Table 60.2

Injury	Lesions of circumflex nerve
Structural impairment	Lesion in continuity – paralysis of deltoid small area of anaesthesia
Subjective impairment	
Disability and handicap	70–85% recovery expected. Recovery takes up to 1 year Little recovery over the age of 50 – such patients permanently handicapped in daily living
Comments	Complication of anterior dislocation of shoulder in 5–18% of cases

Table 60.3

Injury	Lesions of radial nerve (associated with fracture of humerus)
Structural impairment / **Subjective impairment**	Effect of lesion – wrist drop, loss of supination 60% in continuity, with spontaneous recovery (Explore at 8–10 weeks)
Disability and handicap	Use of the hand impeded in complete palsy, as the wrist, thumb and finger joints cannot be extended to allow the hand to clasp an object
Comments	10% incidence with fractures of humeral shaft (Posterior interosseous paralysis can complicate elbow fractures)

Table 60.4

Injury	Division of median nerve at the wrist
Structural impairment / **Subjective impairment**	Loss of sensation over thumb, index, middle and half of ring fingers, and most of palm Paralysis of thenar muscles
Disability and handicap	The disability is severe. Serious disturbance of precision grip compounded by cutaneous anaesthesia. Fine movements and manipulations are impossible (Opposition of the thumb can be restored by tendon transfer)
Comments	The best results of repair restore 70% function Improvement can continue for up to 4 years

Table 60.5

Injury	Division of ulnar nerve at wrist
Structural impairment / **Subjective impairment**	Paralysis of small muscles of hand Loss of sensation over ulnar border of palm, little finger and half ring finger Unimpeded action of long flexors produces characteristic claw hand
Disability and handicap	Loss of power grip. Loss of ability to hold handles of tools (small cylinders). Precision grip also impaired because digits cannot spread to accommodate large objects
Comments	In combined median and ulnar lesions at the wrist, even although the long flexors are spared, the prehensile function of the hand is largely lost and it becomes a simple hook

Compression neuropathies in the upper limb

Tardy ulnar palsy

Most closed lesions of the ulnar nerve occur at the elbow, and some of them, but by no means all, follow injury. The injury, classically to the lateral condyle, can occur in childhood and the palsy may not present clinically for many years. In a review of 110 cases, evidence of childhood fracture was found in 14 (12.7%). Anterior transposition of the nerve produced good results in 85% of the patients in this series (MacNicol, 1979).

Carpal tunnel syndrome

Compression of the median nerve from acute local injury, such as a Colles' fracture, is well recognized. The association of the typical syndrome with injury has been made, usually as repetitive stress. The association is extremely doubtful. Once the diagnosis has been made the carpal tunnel should be decompressed as soon as possible, certainly before motor changes appear. Once they do, they are irreversible (Semple and Cargill, 1969).

References

MacNicol, M. F. (1979) The results of operation for ulnar neuritis. *Journal of Bone and Joint Surgery,* **61B**, 159–164

Semple, J. C. and Cargill, A. O. (1969) Carpal tunnel syndrome. Results of surgical decompression. *Lancet,* **i**, 918–919

Peripheral nerve lesions in the lower limb

Sciatic nerve

The main trunk of the sciatic nerve is vulnerable to injury when the hip is dislocated or the acetabulum is fractured. The lesion is in continuity but spontaneous recovery has been reported as being of the order of 25% of patients (Tile, Kellam and Joyce, 1985). A more optimistic outlook is given by Epstein, who found 11 sciatic nerve lesions in 280 fracture dislocations of the hip. Six of these recovered completely within 30 months (Epstein, 1974).

References

Epstein, H. C. (1974) Posterior fracture dislocations of the hip. *Journal of Bone and Joint Surgery,* **56A**, 1103–1127

Tile, M., Kellam, J. F. and Joyce, M. (1985) Fractures of the acetabulum. *Journal of Bone and Joint Surgery,* **67B**, 324–325

Table 60.6

Injury	Tardy ulnar palsy
Structural impairment / **Subjective impairment**	High lesion in continuity Slow progressive paralysis with symptoms of loss of sensation and pins and needles in little finger, wasting and weakness of small muscles of the hand. Clawing less obvious
Disability and handicap	The disability of an ulnar nerve lesion is slow to appear, and is not as severe as that of the median nerve
Comments	When tardy ulnar palsy is secondary to structural bony abnormality at the elbow, such as childhood fracture, anterior transposition of the nerve gives better results than decompression

The lateral popliteal nerve

The lateral popliteal, or peroneal nerve, is vulnerable on the outer side of the knee, being liable to injury in complications of fractures to the upper tibia and dislocations of the knee. Some traction injuries may inflict complete rupture of the nerve (White, 1968). Being superficial it is easily compressed by tight plaster casts or by the upper edge of a below-knee cast which has been improperly applied. These lesions are in continuity and are expected to recover.

Division of the nerve is found with open wounds. Early suture achieves recovery of motor function in 60–70% of cases. Sensory loss after lateral popliteal division is on the dorsum of the foot and results in little functional disability (Murphey, 1965). The AMA grading for lateral popliteal defect is 38% of the lower limb and 15% of the whole man.

The medial popliteal nerve

The medial popliteal nerve is not as vulnerable as the lateral branch. This is as well because the effects of its division have been compared to those of combined median and ulnar nerve lesions in the hand (Murphey, 1965). The AMA grading for a medial popliteal lesion is 45% impairment of the lower limb and 18% of the whole man. The results of repair are said to be 90% favourable for some recovery of gastrocnemius/soleus function, and between 70% and 80% of patients will recover some pain perception in the foot, thus acquiring some protection against trophic lesions (Murphey, 1965).

References

Murphey, F. (1965) Peripheral nerve injuries. In *Campbell's Operative Orthopaedics* (ed. A. H. Crenshaw), Vol. 2, C. V. Mosby Company, St. Louis, pp. 1538–1582

White, J. (1968) The results of traction injuries to the common peroneal nerve. *Journal of Bone and Joint Surgery,* **50B**, 346–350

Table 60.7

Injury	Closed lesion of sciatic nerve
Structural impairment / **Subjective impairment**	Lesion in continuity. Usually affecting calf and foot Paralysis of calf muscles and small muscles of foot Anaesthesia of foot
Disability and handicap	75% Loss of lower limb function
Comments	25% to 60% Recovery rate. Recovery can occur up to thirty months

Table 60.8

Injury	Closed lesion of lateral popliteal nerve
Structural impairment **Subjective impairment**	Lesion in continuity or complete rupture (Traction injuries) } Drop foot Anaesthesia over small area of dorsum of foot
Disability and handicap	Walking, running, climbing stairs affected Handicap depends on occupation Foot drop controllable by splintage
Comments	If no recovery has begun within 4 months the nerve should be explored Lesions in continuity should recover within 12 months

Part 5

Amputations

61
Amputations

The impairment of an amputation is obvious. The resulting disability or handicap may not be so apparent and can be difficult to assess. The effect of an orthosis in diminishing a handicap will vary widely with the patient's occupation. For example, the handicap imposed by a below-knee amputation stump-fitted with a comfortable patellar tendon bearing limb can be less than that inflicted by a painful, scarred and stiff leg resulting from a severely compound tibial fracture.

The American Medical Association has produced tables for permanent impairment following amputation, as affecting the 'whole man'. They are reproduced here, but should be applied selectively to the individual patient. Most amputation stumps have consolidated within 6 months, although complications of healing, which include adherent scars, neuromata or phantom pain, may persist and imply that prognosis be deferred until they are resolved. The assessment of residual disability and handicap following upper limb amputation should take into account the patient's occupation and the potential of retraining. Assessment of lower limb amputation should include gait analysis with the definitive orthosis. Amputation, particularly in the young adult, inflicts significant psychological trauma in addition to the mutilation. The severity of this mental trauma is often less when the amputation is carried out immediately after the injury than when it is performed after the failure of prolonged surgical reconstruction.

Table 61.1 Impairment following amputations

Amputation	*Percentage impairment of 'whole man'*
Upper limb	
Forequarter amputation	70
Disarticulation at shoulder joint	60
Above-elbow amputation	60
Disarticulation through elbow	57
Below-elbow amputation	54
Disarticulation at wrist joint	54
Midcarpal amputation	54
Amputation of all fingers except thumb at metacarpophalangeal joints	32
Amputation of thumb at metacarpophalangeal joint	22
Amputation of thumb at interphalangeal joint	16
Amputation of index at metacarpophalangeal joint	14
Amputation of index at proximal interphalangeal joint	11
Amputation of index at distal interphalangeal joint	6
Amputation of middle finger at metacarpophalangeal joint	11
Amputation of middle finger at proximal interphalangeal joint	8
Amputation of middle finger at distal interphalangeal joint	5
Amputation of ring finger at metacarpophalangeal joint	5
Amputation of ring finger at proximal interphalangeal joint	4
Amputation of ring finger at distal interphalangeal joint	3
Amputation of little finger at metacarpophalangeal joint	3
Amputation of little finger at proximal interphalangeal joint	2
Amputation of little finger at distal interphalangeal joint	1
Lower Limb	
Hemipelvectomy	50
Disarticulation at hip	40
Above-knee amputation	36
Disarticulation through knee (or Gritti–Stokes amputation)	36
Below-knee amputation	28
Syme's amputation	28
Metatarsophalangeal amputation, all toes	8
Amputation of great toe	8
Amputation of 2nd–5th toe	2

Reproduced with permission from *Guides to the Evaluation of Permanent Impairment*, American Medical Association, 1977.

Index